658. 91362

(2) (5 (2)

Out of
print
July 10.

**Business
Planning
in the
Health
Service**

Business Planning in the Health Service

Peter Jones
*Director-Consultancy, Internal Audit
and Consultancy Services Ltd*

Jonathan Bates
*Deputy Finance Director / Mid-
Kent Healthcare Trust*

INTERNATIONAL THOMSON BUSINESS PRESS
I(T)P An International Thomson Publishing Company

London · Bonn · Boston · Johannesburg · Madrid · Melbourne · Mexico City · New York · Paris
Singapore · Tokyo · Toronto · Albany, NY · Belmont, CA · Cincinnati, OH · Detroit, MI

Business Planning in the Health Service

First published by International Thomson Business Press

A division of International Thomson Publishing Inc.
The ITP logo is a trademark under licence

British Library Cataloguing-in-Publication Data
A catalogue record for this book is available from the British Library

First edition 1996

Typeset by Saxon Graphics Ltd, Derby
Printed in the UK by Cambridge University Press, Cambridge

ISBN 1-86152-020-4

International Thomson Business Press
Berkshire House
168–173 High Holborn
London WC1V 7AA
UK

International Thomson Business Press
20 Park Plaza
14th Floor
Boston MA 02116
USA

http: //www. thomson. com/itbp. html

Contents

Preface

It is an old adage that time spent planning is seldom wasted. No where is this so true as in organisations where problems are complex and the solutions required, novel. This is clearly the situation in today's health service.

One of the key issues that the recent changes in the NHS have attempted to tackle has been the need for strong management – strong management to tackle amongst other things, the demands for higher quality, relentlessly increasing efficiency and modern industrial relations. The changes have sought to achieve improved management by setting up new structures and new accountabilities. The purchaser/provider split is the basic structure, the new management tools are:

- devolved line management responsibilities;
- private sector financial management systems, and
- business/strategic planning methods.

Business planning is therefore one of the major tools that the NHS will use, it is implicit in its new management structure.

Devolved line management, modern financial management and business planning are all techniques that work well together. In all the public services but particularly in health, decision making has been radically devolved to local organisations and decision makers closer to patients and to other health related agencies in the community. The purchaser/provider split, market testing and local fundholding have caused hospitals, community based services, general practitioners and others to plan in detail for *their* patients and customers, while the 'centre' seeks more and more to facilitate rather than to control. This change calls for a new style of planning from all the participants both purchaser and provider.

Business planning is an appropriate management tool for the health service. The NHS is highly complex. Health service organisations have many individual departments – nursing, district nursing, porters, mortuary, health physics, computer services amongst other things. Each has internal and external customers.

The health service is a large number of separate businesses each with their own strategic planning needs. Each department will need to formulate its strategy in its own 'business plan'. Together all the departmental plans will coalesce into a hospital or trust business plan!

Business planning is a flexible management tool; it is highly responsive to these diverse needs and the instability inherent in organisations that are 'demand led' from patients and purchasers. Whatever your initial reaction to business planning, favourable or not, this book will help. It is designed for managers who need to evaluate the approach for the first time and those who are already seeking to maximise its benefit for their organisation.

Chapter 1

Introduction

AIMS OF THE BOOK

This book provides practical guidance for managers in the health service who need to prepare or revise business plans. Although some jargon and theory are unavoidable, we have kept this to a minimum, presenting the reader with something we hope he or she will want to read and use. To help achieve this, case studies are a significant feature of the book.

The public services, in particular the National Health Service (NHS), are required to produce business plans for enterprises that are expected to be businesslike in a broadly commercial sense but do not have the independence and freedom to take full advantage of the free market. A private enterprise regulated by the 1985 Companies Act will, on the whole, be less tightly controlled than any part of the NHS and subjected to few controversial political constraints. The best aspects of business planning have evolved to meet the needs of private enterprise. This means that some selection and adaptation is generally required to make full use of such aspects in the more regulated and politically sensitive environment of health services. This book selects, adapts and innovates best practice to meet the needs of health service readers, although readers from other public services may well find the book useful for their business planning.

Unpredicted reversals in political policy, a constantly shifting regulatory regime and unclear definitions of 'customers' will be familiar concepts to many managers reading this book. Fortunately, this is just the type of uncertain environment in which business planning has already proved useful to a wide range of private and public sector managers.

Since the early 1980s Government initiatives and legislation have combined to transform the structure of the health service in the UK. The NHS and Community Care Act 1990, the Patient's Charter, a wide range of performance indicators issued by the Department of Health and the 'Health of the Nation' report are primary examples. But the most critical development for business planning is the split that has emerged between purchasers and providers or clients and contractors. The large-scale purchasers or clients are the health authorities and GP fundholding practices. The large-scale contractors are hospitals, ambulance services, and various primary and community care bodies. This development has focused minds on the strategic objectives of organizations – and hence on business plans.

Business plans are usually considered from a contractor's viewpoint, but in practice a single body will normally take on both roles to varying extents. For instance, hospitals have the purchasing or client role for agency nurses or catering. The client–contractor split has been an inevitable outcome of the so-called 'internal market' encouraging purchasers and providers to act more competitively, broadly emulating the free market of the private sector. The examples in this book mainly involve contracting situations but the principles apply to purchasing too.

Neither the internal market nor the so-called free market is unregulated and, as we have seen, the same regulations do not necessarily apply to both. New or relatively unfamiliar mechanisms have been introduced to assist competition as one of the broad aims of Government economic policy. Among the most important mechanisms are market testing, including compulsory competitive tendering, and service-level agreements or contracts between clients and contractors. In addition, health care has been opened up to many forms of private sector involvement. These are mechanisms that call for business planning if strategic management is to be effective.

This book seeks to avoid any political side-taking. It simply takes the reality of the situation and provides guidance and some extra tools to enable professional managers to do the best work possible. Although we draw heavily upon the current state of the health service, the principles and methods outlined will remain widely applicable under the different policies currently being put forward by the main political parties.

The requirements of the NHS Executive are considered when appropriate, especially regarding capital business cases in Chapter 8.

However, for specific detail, we suggest that readers turn to the latest 'Executive Letters', manual or other guidance from the NHS. This book seeks to make business planning a useful management tool, rather than follow what is, unfortunately, often seen by managers as a bureaucratic requirement of the NHS.

BACKGROUND KNOWLEDGE REQUIRED

This book is aimed at a wide range of professionals, any of whom may find themselves involved in business planning. We assume no particular specialist knowledge; financial, medical, legal or other. What is assumed is that a business planner will have vision, a lateral thinking mind, will learn quickly and be able to accommodate diverse, sometimes conflicting, views and aspirations. He or she also must not hesitate to pay attention to detail when this is important. This is a tall order, perhaps, but these are the kind of characteristics that will determine the success of the plan.

While particular professional or specialist knowledge is not assumed, ready access to expertise is. The business planner from, say, a general surgery background with some management experience will, we assume, have access to accountants, personnel and other specialists, or be part of a planning team that includes these. Even when the organization is relatively small the advice of external specialist firms and links to other public bodies can be assumed.

Chapter 2

Reasons for business planning

TYPICAL REASONS

There are probably as many reasons for business planning as there are plans or planners. The important point is to be clear about the reasons for the plan that *you* are preparing. Checklist 1 lists some fairly typical broadly worded reasons. Although these tend to have been used with the private sector in mind, such reasons also apply to today's health service. In addition to the reasons shown in Checklist 1, the National Health Service Executive (NHS(E)), requires NHS bodies to prepare a yearly plan, with a summary, for publication.

Checklist 1

Examples of reasons for preparing business plans are:

- The need to convince outside investors to lend finance, such as loans from banks or extended trade credit. In the NHS this will include the Private Finance Initiative (PFI), considered in more detail in Chapter 9.
- To obtain grants of public funds from central or local government.
- As part of preparing a tender bid for a long-term contract. Most contractors will undertake business planning to cater for their major contracts. Many health and other public bodies now face tendering for a single contract upon which the success of their entire business rests.
- As a means of motivating staff at all levels.
- As part of a system of quality management.
- As a coherent framework to guide and measure progress towards planned goals.

- As a marketing tool.
- As a financial planning tool.

LIMITATIONS OF TRADITIONAL HEALTH SERVICE PLANNING

In almost any type of enterprise it will be necessary to plan at a strategic level. In many cases the results of such planning will include elements of business planning, although, as we shall discuss, much traditional health planning and public sector planning elsewhere has revolved around three aspirations:

1. maintaining the organization's *status quo*;
2. dealing with urgent events, often resulting from point 1 above;
3. accommodating to changes in political policy and initiatives.

The health service, funded from taxation, has traditionally been subject to much the same influences of centralized, or centrally controlled, 'state' planning as the rest of the public sector. Attitudes towards planning, both inside and outside the health service, should be seen against this background.

Sometimes these points, particularly the third, may still be relevant to a business plan. But even when they are necessary, they will be far from sufficient. Business plans must aim from the start to cater simultaneously for external as well as internal needs, rather than putting the internal needs first and catering for external pressures when these become irresistible.

In the past, health service deliverers at the hospital or other service providing body have, rightly, planned to maintain or enhance their professional specialisms and the quality of the service they deliver. They could be expected to see their roles almost exclusively as surgeons, nurses, psychologists etc. with a limited amount of management involvement to maintain low level maintenance objectives. Changing professional and administrative needs, broadly classed as 'internal' to the organization itself, were their main concern when planning for change. Changing demographic, environmental, economic and market forces, broadly classed as 'external', were almost exclusively the responsibility of the bureaucracy at regional or national level. This is still partly the situation today, particularly with regard to the Department of Health, the NHS Executive and local health authorities. But individual hospitals, Trusts and business units can no longer leave it to the external bureaucracy, which is the purchasing side of the split referred to earlier, to assess the external factors on their behalf. They must:

- make themselves aware of plans on the purchasing side as soon as possible and start to assess the impact on their own unit's business plan;
- take into account any relevant external factors not considered by the purchasing side or at government department level. Such factors may have been underestimated or missed, or may simply be peculiar to their own unit. This point leads naturally into the next;
- consider ways to compete with other providing units. For most such units the ability to be first in the field by spotting external changes in demand from patients, other client business units and the health service purchasing side will be an important competitive advantage. Even awareness of minor changes in standards and subtle nuances of accepted service provision can offer advantage and increase the general quality and appreciation of service.

For example, a pathology unit may become aware of new analytical methods or a managerial improvement that can increase its efficiency or effectiveness long before any new practice can be assessed and circularized from the level of government or local purchasing bureaucracy. As another example, an ambulance service may become aware of routes and communities that are developing or that it can serve better than the hospital's existing service.

Clearly, local purchasing units will have as much need to increase their awareness of external factors as contracting units. At the same time, neither should underestimate the potential use that can be made of centrally-provided information and services when it comes to, say, bulk purchases, specialized expertise and the dissemination of policy and regulatory information such as European Union (EU) competition requirements.

Clearly, these obligations place a far greater emphasis than in the past on devolved power and decision making. This is why business planning is so important: it allows an organization to achieve more control over, and regulates, its own destiny.

LIMITATIONS OF COMMERCIAL BUSINESS PLANNING

Business planning arises from the need to plan at a strategic level, particularly to meet major commercial objectives in a national or international free market. Objectives in the health service have to take account of the more regulated internal market. Although fundholders can purchase services from several possible suppliers, including suppliers outside the traditional health service units, they do not have total commercial freedom to, say, produce services themselves, thereby negating the purchaser–provider split. Even managers of relatively small business units must learn to think in strategic terms rather than leaving this largely to officials at the national or regional level. Their survival as an economic unit in competition with other units depends upon their own effort and, as we said earlier, their ability to win contracts. Even when their position seems relatively secure, they still need to offer services at a price that will discourage their traditional purchasers from taking their custom elsewhere.

Although such business plans will inevitably be directed by commercial considerations, where services to people are concerned the commercial considerations are not just financial. Any responsible and successful provider of 'people services', such as hotels, banks, leisure services and so on, will be aware that perceptions of quality, status and many other less tangible factors can play a critical part in commercial success. If this is so for banks, hotels and leisure, it is even more the case for health services, where the usual qualitative perceptions of the customer are further complicated by the political dimension, which includes standards and targets set by government and the composition and influence of local political groups. Pressures to respond to the 'politically correct' norms are far more likely to affect the provision of health care than most 'people services' provided in the free market. As a result, many business plans in the health services have already started to take on board these wider social objectives, as we will see from some of the examples and case studies discussed later.

POLITICAL CONSIDERATIONS AND ACCOUNTABILITY

Despite what has been written earlier about traditional state planning and its implied abandonment, health service provision is still of concern to many politicians, electors and pressure groups. Business plans often need to take account of these wider political concerns in different ways.

At a broad level, the basic objectives of a health service body may reflect political aspirations regarding, for example, the length of waiting time for treatment, standards of care, or equal opportunities and access to services. At a narrower level, particular performance criteria may be set, such as the 'Health of the Nation' risk factor targets set by the Government in the early 1990s for the health service as a whole to meet by the year 2000. The objectives of particular business units may need to reflect such 'political' targets if they are to satisfy the purchasing client, particularly if the clients pay for the service with government funds.

Most political targets and wider considerations will be expressed in terms of output measures and objectives, and can be fitted into business plans and specified in contracts. Government policies to reduce waiting lists provides one example, and further examples of such political targets are given in the case studies. Some political measures, such as equal employment opportunities, may be input orientated. However, these will normally apply across the whole spectrum of competing organizations and are unlikely to be a major planning concern once they have been clearly specified in law or contract.

Superimposed political objectives not always favoured at board level, or below, sometimes have to be accepted (often with both politicians and senior managers declaring their support, whatever professional reservations exist or party is in power). It is important to appreciate that the health service can be particularly complex in this respect. Political influences, both national and local, colour objectives at different levels and in different health bodies.

Business planning developed in the private sector has tended to take for granted that an organization is entitled to a high level of confidentiality in its affairs. A typical private business, even a large corporation, can rely on widespread commercial confidentiality. The contents of its annual report and accounts to shareholders are highly dependent on the attitude and openness of its directors. This is quite reasonable when private money, including shareholders' funds, is used and put at risk. People and organizations have a lot of choice about where they invest and can usually withdraw their funds promptly or call on legal safeguards. But public money, collected by law, offers no such choice to opt out or specify particular values unlikely to be held by the public at large. Although business units in the health service may be expected to compete as part of a market, the level of confidentially may well be restricted by the need for accountability of public funds. Checklist 2 gives some examples of potential political concerns for business planners.

Checklist 2

Examples of political considerations that may affect business planning:

- Government-set performance targets.
- Decisions on resource allocation, particularly when the choice is between treatment and support services, research or similar indirect activities.
- Hospital and other front-line service closure.
- The siting of proposed new hospitals or other major expansions.
- Testing and piloting new treatments.
- Hospital security, especially at a local level.
- Local, or locally administered, initiatives, for example, Care in the Community, centres for treatment of AIDS, drug abuse etc.
- Arrangements for selecting contractors from the private sector, particularly if contracts might go overspent and motivate calls for information that the contractor may consider confidential.
- Recruitment practices. Some politicians have encouraged so-called positive discrimination in favour of particular minority groups.

In fact the list, potentially, is enormous. The crucial point is that, unlike most commercial business planning, health service plans will be likely to need to take into account politically sensitive issues.

WHY BUSINESS PLANS SOMETIMES FAIL

Without being in any way negative, awareness of the most likely pitfalls is helpful. In Checklist 3 some of the more common ones are cited. They are not in any order of priority.

Checklist 3

Examples of causes of business plan failure:

Internal causes:

- Weak support from management.

- Inability to agree stated aims and objectives.
- Inability to 'harmonize' objectives for different levels or parts of the organization.
- Inability to instil in others the agreed/desired objectives: key people continue to work to their own 'hidden' agenda.
- Poor management and financial information, particularly on clinical activity, costs, commitments and cash flow.
- Poor timing, particularly of restructuring and reorganization.
- Too much or too little detail, resulting in failure to maintain the attention and understanding of the intended audience.
- Failure to involve people and/or match their involvement to their role and potential within the business unit.

External causes:

- Poor timing, particularly in the provision of new or improved services, for example meeting yesterday's needs today.
- Poor management information, particularly market research on customer needs and the actions of competitors.
- Failure to anticipate large-scale changes in demand on a level that is difficult to accommodate, e.g. the closure of major employers and removal of the population base.
- Regulatory changes not envisaged in the plan; for example, EU working hours conditions may prove difficult for some units.

Clearly one could expand these examples. The critical point is to stimulate vision and forethought at the very beginning of the planning process. Where plans have failed they should be analysed and the relevant executives asked to comment on what went wrong.

CONCLUDING POINTS

Although there are many reasons for undertaking business planning, it is important to tailor the plan to the special needs of the health service, rather than simply ape commercial stereotypes. The modern health service needs to match resources to aims and priorities in the most efficient and effective way, and business planning offers a tried and tested method of achieving this.

CASE STUDY 1   WHY HAVE BUSINESS PLANS?

Obstetrics and Gynaecology/Paediatrics (OGP) Directorate, Oak Tree Acute NHS Trust

In this case study we see how a clinical directorate begins to produce a business plan for itself. The senior members of the directorate are meeting and trying to sketch out the major issues they have to consider.

Conrad Campbell, the gynaecologist clinical director of the directorate, is waiting for the rest of the OGP directorate senior personnel to arrive. While reading the business plan for the whole Trust for the first time, he notices that, although OGP represents about 15% of the Trust, it is mentioned only once, as a statistic for the number of babies born each year. It then strikes him that he is not quite sure what else could or should have been included: his strong views on surgical practice are hardly the stuff of business plans. Nevertheless, he had hoped for a little more.

The nurse manager, Cherry Parsons, and the senior paediatrician consultant, Dr Norman Potter, arrive, and Norman asks Conrad what he knows about business plans. 'Not much, except that we don't seem to be included,' is Conrad's reply. Norman approves of this: 'Jolly good thing too. We will be getting profit shares soon.' The group is completed by the arrival of the directorate general manager, Michael Farr, and the management accountant, Pravin Sengupta. Conrad, as chair of the meeting, explains that he has been asked by the chief executive to produce a business plan for the directorate. The Trust produces a corporate business plan each year, as required by the NHS Executive at Quarry House. The meeting was convened by a memo setting out the background issues as seen by the chief executive. Conrad asks Michael to set out his understanding of what is required.

Michael, who had recently moved from a Trust that prided itself on its business planning, comments that the Trust business plan should represent the component directorates that make it up, so 'we need to have clear strategic thoughts of our own, which when added to those of the other six clinical directorates will form a coherent whole.'

Cherry, picking up on the idea of 'strategic' planning, adds 'Our strategy needs to support or at least avoid any conflict with the Trust's wider plans. Presumably ours should also take into account the plans of other directorates?' Michael, while acknowledging this point as one of the main issues, emphasizes that the plan should also be achievable, and not just 'dreamed up' by the chief executive. Cherry and Michael agree that there needs to be communication between the senior management and directorate management. Conrad summarizes this as, 'we are concerned with "strategic planning" and "communication" of the strategic plan both up and down the organization.'

At this point Pravin comments that he has never really thought of OGP as having any strategic planning. Conrad believes that this has been a major problem, causing OGP to 'drift'. He identifies three factors that must be made clear: 'First, what we think we should be trying to achieve in OGP, second, why and, third, when.' Pravin comments that in order to communicate, 'you need to have something to say.'

The meeting concludes with a suggestion from Michael that those present should each give their view of the long-term hopes for the directorate.

Key Learning Points

1. Business planning sets a **strategic context** for work.
2. A key aim of business planning is clarifying and **communicating** objectives.
3. Communication must be both within the **whole organization** and in **individual departments**.
4. Good business planning **harmonizes** the objectives of the organization as a whole, the departments and individuals.

Chapter 3

Business planning and objectives

STRATEGIC OBJECTIVES

The need to plan at the strategic level makes it imperative to consider and clarify strategic objectives. Mission statements, which are discussed in more detail in Chapter 5, are strategic objectives which embody bold statements of purpose. Strategic objectives must be at the forefront of the business plan. Examples are given in Checklist 4.

Checklist 4

Examples of strategic objectives:

- improving particular services;
- raising quality standards;
- increasing market share;
- financial return on assets employed in the business;
- profitability;
- achieving a major capital project.

In any organization strategic objectives must be further broken into various levels of management or operational objectives, according to the structures of different business units and over different time scales.

A HIERARCHY OF OBJECTIVES

It is essential to consider business plans in the context of the hierarchy of organizational objectives. Just as the corporate objectives and mission statements must be backed up by lower order objectives at the level of business units, so any organization-wide business plan must be backed up by appropriate plans at each level. Theoretically, the path to attain a single set of objectives can be achieved in a single business plan. In practice this is mostly possible only in small organizations. Most health services are provided by large organizations in cooperation with other organizations, and even if comprehensive objectives can be agreed, which is often difficult, business planning for units within the larger organizations will usually be essential.

Management objectives might include, for example, reducing the length of a particular waiting list or improving quality control systems to the level of widely recognized quality certification such as ISO 9000 (BS 5750). Such objectives may well vary for each level of management hierarchy. For a simplified example see Figure 1, where the strategic objective is to increase the share of the available market.

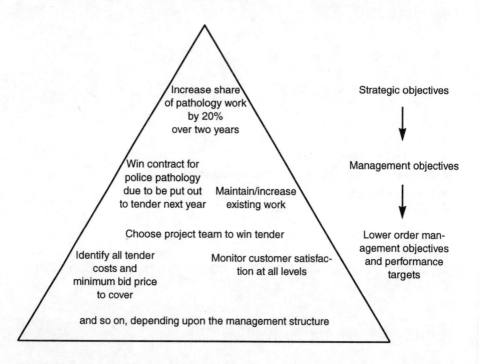

Figure 1 A hierarchy of objectives

HARMONIZATION OF OBJECTIVES

One of the greatest practical difficulties faced in this situation is ensuring that all departmental business plans are in harmony and that different parts of the organization are not wasting efforts and resources or even working against one another. It is possible to produce documents that show various objectives in several business plans, all of which appear to work towards agreed organization-wide strategies; but if these objectives are not being satisfied – and this is almost certain to be so to some extent – pinpointing the objectives that need revision or the deficiencies in the business plans designed to meet the objectives is often a daunting exercise. Indeed, the very appearance of harmony of objectives may be deceiving in the first place. As will be considered later, one of the perennial problems in any planning scenario is the presence of hidden, usually personal, agendas containing powerful objectives that can run counter to the stated 'mission' or to 'local' objectives. Senior corporate management need to work hard to encourage 'good congruence' within the organization.

DEVELOPMENT AND MAINTENANCE OBJECTIVES

It is often useful to distinguish between those objectives aimed at ensuring the smooth continuation of routine work – 'maintenance' objectives – and those designed to fulfil new goals and accommodate change – 'development' objectives. The mission statement (see Chapter 5) and high level objectives need to be explicit about development objectives while still implying the neccessary maintenance objectives. See Checklist 5.

Checklist 5

Examples of maintenance/development type objectives:

Maintenance objectives:

- To fill all nursing staff vacancies within one month.
- To clean all wards to the satisfaction of ward sisters and patients.
- To deal promptly with all emergency admissions.

Development objectives:

- Objectives involving achievement of new or higher standards of treatment.

- The successful completion of a major expansion of facilities.
- To be recognized as a centre of excellence.

Maintenance objectives therefore tend to relate to standards of everyday performance, and development objectives to longer-term vision. Clearly, if a vital maintenance function of the organization cannot be guaranteed then its developmental objectives will not be achieved. Both types are critically important but developments tend to be seen as more prestigious. No doubt greater creativity is associated with vision and change compared to attention to routine detail, past experience and continuing operations. Yet a creative review of familiar operations, such as accommodation charges, can often be more useful by, say, releasing cash to further an organization-wide objective of increasing the number of beds. Conversely, lack of attention to detail has been the downfall of many a new development.

 The critical point is that all of the skills and attributes of a good business planner mentioned in Chapter 1 are likely to count.

CRITICAL CHARACTERISTICS

Some readers may find this emphasis on objectives ironically reminiscent of old-fashioned state planning. Simply making sure that all divisions meet agreed progress towards production quotas with none of the divisional managers stepping seriously out of line is hardly conducive to the sensitive, multipurpose provision of a modern health service. Nothing could be more misleading. Certainly elements of the business planning process will be familiar to planners from any background. The critical differences are freedom, flexibility, fulfilment and/or failure. These arise from the need to respond to customers/clients external to the planning body rather than to internal or appointed, usually political, masters. See Checklist 6.

Checklist 6

Critical characteristics of business planning:

- Freedom, to control the budget and business-related decisions.
- Flexibility, to respond rapidly to the changing needs of customers/clients.
- Fulfilment, by meeting the agreed needs of customers/clients and being rewarded.

- Failure, by not meeting the needs of customers/clients and not being rewarded.

Having the freedom and flexibility means being held solely responsible for the fulfilment or failure. The business unit will be accountable for performance in a way that makes excuses for failure, however understandable, of no concern to the customer or anyone else outside the unit. The consequences will be suffered in isolation or largely so. Customers and clients will be ready to find other suppliers of the service, and likewise suppliers will be ready to seek out new purchasers. Clearly, as business relationships and interdependencies mature, the situation just described can become more complex. Customers will, for example, want to help a key supplier upon which they have come to depend, but only up to a point. The basic situation is far removed from traditional state planning, where a designated planning unit can expect to continue almost irrespective of performance and only selected individuals within the unit may not be rewarded. Of course, selected individuals within a business unit may also not be rewarded but their individual performance can directly determine the rewards or otherwise of colleagues.

INPUT AND OUTPUT MEASURES

Objectives for business plans will usually be set in a way that enables output measures to be used in judging the success of the business unit. Input measures may still matter for internal management purposes such as cost accounting and staffing. But, because the customers/clients are interested in output, the objectives that must be met to remain in existence are output ones and these must be used to formulate the business plan. See Checklists 7 and 8.

Checklist 7

Typical examples of input measures:

- Number of hours worked.
- Cost of wages, salaries and other labour costs per hour, week, month etc., possibly broken down into type of service or department.

- Cost of various drugs or other materials per treatment, time period etc.
- Overhead charges of various types, such as property rentals, utility costs etc.

Checklist 8

Typical examples of output measures:

- Number of operations performed per time period, by type etc.
- Number or proportion of successful operations performed per time period, by type etc.
- Number of chargeable consultancy events per time period, type of activity etc.
- Income generated per activity, unit of output etc.

Clearly, the nature of the business unit and the demands of its customers will determine the precise wording of such measures. Further examples will become apparent in the detailed case studies.

One unit's output may, of course, be another unit's input and the classification of measure between 'input' and 'output' may change as circumstances change.

For example, statistical breakdowns of the number of new surgical dressings per week may be an input measure statistic to an accident unit but an output measure to a central sterile supplies unit. Similarly accounting information will form part of the finance department's output but will be used to measure input costs for many of the front-line service units.

Quite often it is worth going a step further in defining output measures by relating these directly to performance, usually in terms of management objectives or the mission statement. Thus, it will be useful not simply to monitor the number or percentage of, say, successful operations but to relate this to an objective involving, say, comparison with other service providers. Some possible examples are outlined in Checklist 9.

Checklist 9

Examples of output measures related to performance/management objectives:

- To be in the top quartile of surgical units in terms of the numbers of successful operations of a particular type.

- To have the highest success rate for a particular type of treatment anywhere in the UK, for the forthcoming year, for patients of a particular age range.
- To meet the output performance criteria for treatments as set out in a contract, e.g. number of treatments per period, success rate etc.
- To generate a specified level of income or a specified rate of return on capital employed.

The league tables published annually are examples of the importance attached by Government and the Audit Commission to output comparisons. As with all output measures and performance targets or objectives, the nature of the business unit and its clients' needs will determine the precise wording of the measures and objectives.

CONCLUDING POINTS

Without clear and coordinated objectives achievements will be patchy at best. Objectives at each management level and between all parts of a health service body need to be in harmony and focused upon achieving the organization's purposes.

CASE STUDY 2   HIGH LEVEL OBJECTIVES

Obstetrics and Gynaecology/Paediatrics (OGP) Directorate, Oak Tree Acute NHS Trust

Having discussed the benefits of business planning, the management team of the OGP directorate at Oak Tree Acute NHS Trust had decided to set out some of the objectives of the department. Conrad Campbell, the clinical director, is chairing the meeting. The participants express their long-term hopes for the directorate in the following terms:

- Conrad: 'to improve the care we give to older women so that their quality of life is as high as possible.'
- Norman: 'to allow all the sick children we see to reach adulthood so that they can lead normal lives.'
- Cherry: 'to provide first class care to patients and support to parents and the other carers of the very wide range of people we care for.'

- Pravin: 'it is important that we work within budget and do our best to increase income whenever possible.'

This last objective provoked some amusement, but Pravin defended himself by stressing that it is essential to work within the available resources. Failure to do so will result in plans not being implemented properly and 'the Chief Executive will want heads to roll because of the unchecked spending'. Some members of the group, however, still felt that keeping in budget is not an end in itself.

After this exchange, Michael Farr, the general manager, set out his view on an objective and there followed a general discussion on the strengths and weaknesses of the directorate and possibilities for the future. Towards the end of this discussion Michael felt that it would be useful to pull together the threads of the argument:

> 'We have set out a large number of possible aims for the directorate ranging from very broad aspirations to quite specific issues. Norman's first aim was "to allow all the sick children we see to reach adulthood so that they can lead normal lives." But we all had a number of very specific aims. For instance, Cherry wanted to reduce infection rates after surgery by 50%. There are four points to make here. First, let's call our aims "objectives" – they are the objectives we want to achieve as a directorate; second, let's classify our objectives into two types – high level strategic ones and low level operational ones. High level objectives will be broad objectives such as Norman's and operational objectives will be the more specific ones such as Cherry's point on infection. The third point is consistency of objectives. It is vital that we ensure that all the things we want to do really do further the real ends of the directorate and the Trust as a whole. The fourth point is to formulate the objectives in a way that makes it possible to measure achievement in a meaningful way.'

Cherry interprets this as meaning that achievements are presented in terms of the output of services as opposed to inputs, and gives an example related to the obstetrics department:

> 'If we said an objective was to devote all our time and energy to delivering babies we could simply look at our

diaries and say we have achieved our objectives. But if more mothers suffered unnecessary complications than should, or mothers disliked the way we looked after them we would hardly be doing what the public expected of us. It is not what we put in that matters but what we get out. Our objectives should reflect what we consider to be commitments to success, in numerical terms if possible.'

A low level objective in this case might be being in the best 25% of hospitals for perinatal mortality.

Michael comments that for complex issues to be considered in depth, things need to be broken down into 'digestible chunks', to enable efforts to be focused effectively. The idea of a high level objective aids in this process. It is a fundamental objective of an organization. The test is that if such an objective fails to be met, then that organization is likely to cease functioning. Thus, one of the high level objectives of Cherry's unit must be 'to deliver babies' because 'if we didn't we wouldn't be an obstetrics department'. Michael comments that, although it may seem like stating the obvious, it is important that the high level objectives are made explicit, for two major reasons:

'First, organizations often forget what their real reasons for existence are. For instance, before I became directorate manager here my work involved some property management duties. Until about 15 years ago many central heating boilermen in large buildings thought that polishing the brasswork was an important objective. They never thought that no one ever looked at it and polishing served no maintenance function. Second, even if high level objectives are very clear and well understood we need to state them so that we are able to check that our operational objectives further our high level ones. It is surprising how often people's operational objectives bear no relation to their strategic ones.'

The participants agree to put their high level objectives down on paper.

High level objectives of the OGP directorate

1. To deliver babies safely, providing the highest quality care to children and mothers.

2. To provide the best quality medical care to women suffering from reproductive medical conditions.
3. To strive to ensure that sick children reach adulthood so that they can lead normal lives.
4. To ensure that all Patient's Charter requirements are met.

Conrad had fought hard for another objective, 'that all medical and nursing staff receive the best opportunities for training', but the others spent 10 minutes trying to explain that this objective was a secondary one, which would help the achievement of the primary ones. Good training would be required to help ensure that sick children reached adulthood. As Pravin put it, 'you may find it surprising, but doctors are just a symptom of an imperfect world.'

Another suggested high level or primary objective was that 'links with primary care teams in the community should be strengthened'. After discussion, it was agreed that this too was an operational objective. However, this objective was much less clearly of a operational nature because current health policy puts such great stress on this major change in the way care is provided. Norman had said that unless they achieved this objective the OGP directorate would receive reduced funding from the local health authority and their survival as a strong directorate would at some stage be in doubt. Cherry and Conrad disagreed, saying that better primary care links would just be another way of achieving their other primary objectives of best care to women and children. In fact, this objective could arguably have been included in either category.

By this stage the meeting had produced some useful results. They decided that another should be convened in a week's time to set out operational objectives and pull together the major components of a business plan for the directorate. The participants were requested to bring a set of operational objectives for discussion to this meeting.

Key Learning Points

1. Objectives are usefully classified into two categories: **high level** (or primary) and **operational** (or secondary).
2. High level objectives are the **fundamental aims** of a department or organization. If they fail to be met, the department or organization is likely to fail.

3. High level objectives relate to **organizational outputs** not inputs or processes.
4. **Written analysis** of objectives encourages clarification of what is essentially important to an organization or department.

CASE STUDY 3 OPERATIONAL OBJECTIVES

Obstetrics and Gynaecology/Paediatrics (OGP) Directorate Oak Tree Acute NHS Trust

Second meeting

When the management team met again the following week, Michael started by further explaining business planning as he saw it.

'If any organization is going to be successful it needs to plan from very broad objectives through to doing specific useful things. In order to cure children we need high quality staff, up-to-date equipment, effective training and good links with GPs. To move to the next stage, to have, say, effective training we need to identify what training will be "effective" – what courses do we need? Who provides them? When are they available? Lastly, we need to agree the training with staff, book the courses and pay for them. There is therefore a hierarchy between the very broad objective, moving down to a whole range of very specific actions. The business plan sets out these objectives and links the actions needed to fulfil them so that what we do is properly thought through.'

This analysis received the grudging acceptance of all participants. It all seemed rather long winded but there was little that could be objected to. At this point each person set out his or her operational objectives for the directorate. The ideas of the clinical director, the senior consultant and the nursing manager are set out below:

Conrad Campbell, clinical director:

1. New obstetrics operating theatre for Caesarean sections.
2. Research project trialing new methods of minimizing female surgery.

3. Work towards a goal of cutting infection rates after surgery by 50% in three years.
4. Training for medics of all grades in the directorate in up-to-date best practice.
5. Work towards identifying 50% more of the abnormalities in children born under the directorate's care.

Norman Potter, senior consultant:

1. Set up a centre of paediatric excellence for the area.
2. Work towards a goal of reducing child deaths after birth by 50% in five years.
3. Set up research work monitoring long-term success of children born before 32 weeks of pregnancy.
4. Agree and put in place a code of practice for the care of children and adolescents.

Cherry Parsons, nursing manager:

1. Change grade structure of nursing department to ensure that all staff are paid at an acceptable level.
2. Work towards improving the role of midwives in the birth experience.
3. Improve the facilities for new mothers in the hospital.

When the objectives had been read out Michael suggested that they try to link them to the high level or primary objectives that had been devised at the previous meeting. For example, the idea of a special theatre for Caesarean sections would presumably help the achievement of primary objective 1, 'delivering babies safely'. Under the existing arrangement, the OGP directorate has to request a theatre from the surgery directorate when the need arises, which, as Conrad pointed out, 'makes us horribly dependent on them'. Norman, however, objected that such situations occur infrequently, and 'in any event you would still need their anaesthetists and theatre nurses'.

Pravin Sengupta, the management accountant, gave his assessment of the suggestion:

'A new theatre would cost at least £200 000. The capital charges excluding any increased running costs for the directorate would be £20 000 a year or the cost of 30 routine operations. Conrad, I'm afraid your objective is in the category of boilermen polishing brasswork. It does not satisfy a high level objective – but it does satisfy you!'

After this, Conrad's objective of an additional theatre was dropped. His other objectives were agreed and linked to primary objectives as follows:

2. Research project trialing new methods of minimizing female surgery: *primary objective 2.*
3. Work towards a goal of cutting infection rates after surgery by 50% in 3 years: *primary objective 2.*
4. Training for medics of all grades in the directorate in up-to-date best practice: *primary objectives 1, 2 and 3.*
5. Work towards identifying 50% more abnormalities in children born under the directorate's care: *primary objectives 1 and 3.*

Moving on to Norman's objectives, the first, *to set up a centre of paediatric excellence for the area*, was again contentious although they all started by agreeing that this was an excellent idea. Oak Tree Acute Trust could have its paediatric specialty as a leader in care nationally. This would clearly meet primary objective 3 and help in meeting objective 1. Again, though, it was Pravin who started to object:

'I think that we are making a mistake here. We are falling into the boilerman syndrome again. We all like the idea of a paediatric centre of excellence, it makes us all feel good. The problem is, how are we going to fund it?'

According to Norman, if it is a centre of excellence more children will be referred. Success will breed success. Pravin, however, argued that:

'That is not how it will work unless we convince our purchasers. What would our main purchaser, the local health authority, think? Have you asked them? They will not send us extra patients unless it fits with their strategic planning about where they see centres of local excellence.'

Norman's view is that the OGP directorate has a good specialty, which should be built up to benefit patients further: 'If they, the local health authority, don't accept that argument then all our suspicions about purchaser–provider splits will be confirmed'. This view, however, cuts little ice with the management accountant:

'Our suspicions might be confirmed and your pride crushed but that is probably the only local issue. We believe we should be a centre of paediatric excellence because we like the idea. The health authority as a major purchaser would not see it so personally. They would look at current centres of excellence – for instance, Ranborne Trust, just 25 miles away. They would look at areas where there are large numbers of children and a high birth rate – certainly not here, where we have a high level of retired people. But, even more importantly, we need to find out about their strategic planning. I believe that if they were likely to have us in their strategic plan they would have been talking to us already.'

The participants agreed that Pravin had a point: It was no use having grandiose plans unless the patients could be guaranteed, and that meant talking to purchasers.

After this exchange, it was agreed that Norman and the Trust contracts director would approach the local health authority, the other large health authority purchasers and the GP fundholders to see if they had strategic plans or long-term views on paediatric and obstetric and gynaecology needs so that the directorate business plan could be tied in with their medium-term ideas.

Norman's remaining objectives and those of Cherry were agreed, with the exception of Cherry's proposal to change the grade structure of the nursing department. Although they all agreed that it would be nice to pay nurses more, without a recruitment or quality problem this was not going to satisfy a primary objective.

Michael summarized as follows:

'We have all produced a set of practical operational objectives, which could be implemented in the medium term. The question is, though, are these objectives important to our organization? Have we covered the major areas for which we have a professional responsibility? I would say we clearly have not. I don't mean more detail: I mean, in some ways, the opposite. For example, one of Norman's four objectives was to monitor children's success. This is 25% of his objectives but will probably take about 1% of his specialty's time. What he has not included as an objective is doing well what he does most of his day, i.e. seeing patients.'

He went on to stress that it is useful to divide the business plan objectives into two categories, maintenance objectives and development objectives. The participants had so far concentrated almost entirely on the latter, but, as Conrad pointed out, 'We have to plan to maintain the service as well as develop it. Even the *status quo* doesn't happen by itself. It requires daily grind'. An example of a maintenance requirement would be to continue to deliver babies in best practice conditions to the satisfaction of mothers and the benefit of children. This sets a number of clear standards – 'best practice', 'satisfaction' and 'benefit' – which are all things that to a greater or lesser extent can be measured or monitored, once the standards have been set: Outputs need to be measured against agreed criteria to enable monitoring of the quality and quantity of the work. When Pravin pointed out that monitoring was not made clear in the objective, Michael reminded him that the meeting had started with a discussion of the business planning *hierarchy*.

Key Learning Points

1. Operational objectives must **link** directly to specific high level objectives.
2. Operational objectives must be **practical**. They should be linked with perceived organizational strengths (ideally as set out in a SWOT analysis; see Case Study 6).
3. In the health service it is important always to consider the likely **views of purchasers**.
4. Objective setting should **avoid excessive detail** since this will obscure the message. Objectives should not exceed two pages of A4.
5. Operational objectives can usefully be divided into two categories, **maintenance** and **development**.
6. Objectives must be set precisely so that they clearly cover both **quality** and **quantity** issues.

CASE STUDY 4   THE BUSINESS PLANNING HIERARCHY

Obstetrics and Gynaecology/Paediatrics (OGP) directorate, Oak Tree Acute NHS Trust

The next meeting of the business planning group of the OGP directorate, attended by Michael Farr, Conrad Campbell and Pravin Sengupta, considered the business planning hierarchy further. Recapping on the previous meeting, Michael said:

'We need to think about objectives before we think about doing specific tasks. As we have discussed, objectives can be classified as "high level" and "operational", so we get a hierarchy of high level objectives; operational objectives; specific tasks.'

Pravin pointed out that 'there is a level below tasks – namely, budgets'. To begin with, though, they considered the simple hierarchy. The hierarchy links high level objectives to pounds sterling. It is the core of the business planning process. In the public sector this link is especially vivid. Parliament passes an Act requiring the delivery of health care to the people; it then passes a yearly Finance Act to ensure that the money is there to allow the health care to be delivered. Parliament can relatively easily set the broad policy objectives and vote the money; what it cannot do is ensure that the money is spent *productively* on meeting those objectives, hence the whole public debate on public sector waste and reorganization of 'business' units. All of the changes are at least based on trying to make sure that money does lead to health care.

What Conrad finds interesting about this is the need for a clear chain of 'events' linking objectives to people writing cheques: 'It is very easy to ignore this necessary progression and just get on with the daily round'. Pravin recalled an example of failure of this 'chain' from his time as an auditor in local government:

'When controls over local authority capital spending came in, no council wanted to waste its allocation. For some authorities the allocation was in fact considerably higher than they normally spent. The result was that some had enormous capital programmes which each year were solemnly approved by councillors but were never achieved. This went on for several years until the allocations were cut back.'

These authorities had detailed objectives which were not linked 'down' to clear tasks and were probably not linked 'up' to coherent high level objectives. The major problem was that their objectives were incomplete. They knew what schemes they wanted to do – these were valid operational objectives. However, a whole range of other operational objectives had not been identified, nor were the operational objectives set to support policy or strategic objectives, other than simply to divert funds from central to local government. As a result, all of the requirements for professional staffing, training and management, or contracting out of these functions, had not been tackled. There was a great gap in the objectives covering all that side of things, with the result that the links mentioned above were not in place, the outcome being that even with money little was achieved. This is why it is so important that the business planning hierarchy is set down clearly in writing, so that a complete and coherent view is taken.

Putting this analysis in the context of the OGP directorate, Conrad said:

'We set high level objectives which are our fundamental aims. We then set operational objectives that satisfy the high level objectives. We do this, making sure that we have been as practical as we can be. It is critical to ensure that the secondary objectives taken as a whole will allow us to achieve the high level objectives. Then we set out those tasks we need to achieve to meet the operational objectives. Lastly, we spend the money that Parliament, via purchasers, has given us to carry out the task!'

Using the OGP directorate as an example, part of the hierachy can be illustrated as follows:

- High level objective: to deliver babies safely, providing the highest quality care to children and mothers.
- Operational objective: training for clinical staff of all disciplines and grades in the directorate in up-to-date best practice.
- Task: identify training needs and send staff on appropriate courses on a timely basis.
- Cost: Training budget of £7500.

In fact, for a whole department there is a web of interrelating objectives, tasks and budgets. The operational objective relating to training for clinical staff will also apply to some of the other high level objectives that were identified, such as 'to provide the best quality medical care to women suffering from reproductive medical conditions' (see Case Study 2). The concept of training is a particularly straightforward example of how the hierarchy looks: training expenditure has a simple and linear link to the high level objective. Many objectives are more complicated. For example, in a service industry the staff do nearly everything. As a result, staffing represents the majority of the costs at one end of the hierarchy and the staff meet most of the high level objectives at the other. The issue of staff therefore needs to be broken down into component elements. The staff budget must be spent on a selection of personnel who are optimal in the circumstances. Pravin illustrated the practical problems associated with this as follows:

'If an objective is to reduce infection after surgery, how does this affect staffing and costs? Much more complicated planning will obviously be needed. For instance, one might need to change ward layouts and this might affect the nursing staff skill mix needed. In addition, a skill mix to meet an infection objective might not be optimal for some of the other aims of the directorate.'

Key Learning Points

1. The hierarchy is the **core** of the business planning process, ensuring that money is spent on tasks that will achieve identified objectives.
2. In the health service the link between budgets and high level objectives is clearly set out within the **Parliamentary process**.
3. Business planning is effective only if the hierarchy is complete. **Incomplete links** within the hierarchy will cause problems. Just as importantly, **incompletely identified** objectives, tasks or budgets will damage the process.
4. Because business planning is relatively complex, it is important that it is **well documented** to aid clarification of the steps and identification of opportunities.
5. **Staffing** is a particularly important part of business planning in health and service industries.

Chapter 4

The business planning process

BASIC FRAMEWORK

Although the contents of business plans vary enormously, we now need to consider a fairly typical practical framework, a basic outline or model. The limitations of our basic outline will become apparent as we progress. But without such a framework it would be more difficult to understand and appreciate the complex practicalities and possible variations that are considered later and required in practice.

The framework is presented in a simplified form in Figure 2 with typical headings in Checklist 10. More detailed attention is given in later chapters to mission statements, marketing, finance and other key areas.

Checklist 10

Typical headings:

- Introduction: background to the body and the planned achievements.
- High level statements: mission, strategy, purpose, future aims etc.
- Services/products: descriptions of what the organization provides.
- Objectives: at various levels, from senior management to work targets.
- Market: main purchasers/customers, new services, expansion etc.
- Personnel: people involved and personnel management policy.

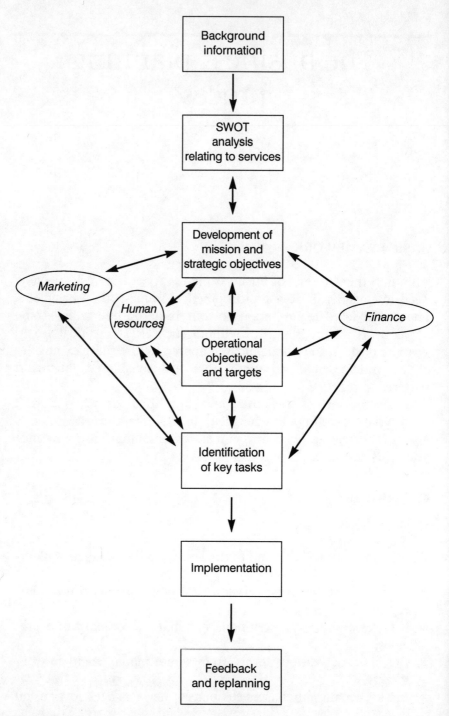

Figure 2 A business planning process model

- Finance: past performance, new sources of funding, etc.
- Major schemes: capital expansion, recruitment initiatives, new IT etc.

Three points should be borne in mind when considering the above framework:

1. The figure and the checklist both present a rather rigid impression of business planning. In any situation the stages adopted will suit the organization's specific needs even though the final plan may contain the elements outlined above.
2. Business plans should be updated frequently in almost any organization.
3. All headings will not necessarily have equal importance either in relation to the other headings or in relation to different business units in the same organization. In practice, many plans appear to concentrate on one or two headings, such as marketing or finance. This concentration is usually either because the high level statements are dominated by, say, financial or marketing aspirations, or because the main purpose in drawing up the plan was to attract finance, expand the business unit etc.

Let us now consider some of the areas in a little more detail.

BACKGROUND INFORMATION

This heading might cover the development and history of the organization or business unit, the broad type of services provided, key achievements and relationships to other local and national bodies. Broad policy objectives might be implied, but not usually in detail as these will be more explicitly formulated and outlined as high level statements.

This part of the plan should be kept as short as possible. Most readers of business plans will not be greatly concerned with background details. At the same time, however, such introductory aspects can be critical in winning readers over to the organization's broad sentiments and encourage them to approach the rest of the plan in a positive frame of mind.

HIGH LEVEL STATEMENTS AND STRATEGIC OBJECTIVES

Many terms are used to describe these statements – vision

statements, strategic policy, board level objectives – but the most widely used term is 'mission statements'. Usually they determine, and may be indistinguishable from, major objectives. They are in fact that part of the plan that contains the basic rationale and key aims of the business. It is difficult to avoid tautology when defining such high level statements. They are above tactical and most managerial level objectives and may be implied rather than explicit. In the health service, mission statements are likely to contain more varied sentiments and purposes than most private sector commercial business plans. This reflects the wider social aims of the service. These may sometimes sound unbusinesslike on first reading, although further consideration will usually reveal a depth of thought required to combine commercial and social considerations into a single mission. Examples of mission statements and more detailed discussion of this aspect of the plan are given in Chapter 5. It is vital to produce high level statements that are up to date and genuinely reflect the realistic aims of the service.

MANAGEMENT OBJECTIVES AND SERVICES

Figure 2 mentions operational objectives and targets and, as in Checklist 10, a heading exists for services. Various terms are used for objectives at different levels of management to suit the structure of the body concerned: senior management objectives, management objectives, operational objectives, performance targets etc. In practice, these are closely bound up with the services provided, and in business planning it is almost impossible to consider services without management objectives or vice versa.

By this stage the planning process will have identified services and products, relating them to different customers, groups of patients or purchasers. The management/operational objectives will be set to satisfy patient and purchaser needs. At this stage in particular (and throughout the planning process in general) it is important to ensure that such lower level objectives are clearly related to the mission and strategic objectives. This is considered in more detail in Chapter 5.

Departments and business units within the organization should 'own' a set of objectives and services. Although slight overlap of services is not unusual, perhaps when one unit provides a specialized stage of a wider service, significant duplication of effort within the same organization is usually inefficient. For example, paramedics may perform a holding treatment on an accident victim before admission to a surgical ward, but two separate payroll units would need to be questioned!

Overlapping objectives are common and, indeed, to be expected if the organization has a clear and easily adopted mission statement. All business units may, for example, set operational objectives of attaining defined quality standards as part of their route to fulfilling a mission statement that includes quality of service.

Clearly, a good business plan will cover all operations that can have an impact upon the mission statement. A summary of the plan, or at least of the services and objectives, is often convenient for external readers, the work-force or anyone not deeply involved in the planning process. The detail may well have an element of confidentiality, although in the health service any confidentiality will need to be gauged against issues of public interest, considered on page 9.

Targets and future aspects of the different services and business units may conveniently be included in this part of the plan, although some planners may prefer to include these aspects under marketing.

Comparisons over time and with other similar health service bodies may also fall naturally into this part of the plan, although, once again, marketing or possibly finance may be the practical 'home' for such comparisons.

PEOPLE AND HUMAN RESOURCES

Business plans can provide a useful opportunity to inspire confidence in the work-force of an organization at all levels. The part of the plan dealing with human resources is usually an ideal opportunity to achieve this. As a minimum, short biographies of senior managers should be included. The human resources of the organization can be compared to the operational objectives. It is particularly useful when large numbers of staff are involved to stress the training and career development policy and practices, showing how these enhance the business.

The planning process will need to tackle the often complex issues involved in managing human resources to meet targets and objectives, particularly in respect of major projects. Capital works, information technology and other major projects are often of a 'one-off' nature, making human resource needs particularly difficult to plan in advance. The skills and availability of staff at a cost that can be afforded will usually need to be given as much attention as financial, property, material and other resources. Chapter 7 discusses human resources in more detail.

Checklists 11 and 12 give examples of some of the people attributes and policy areas that contribute to this part of the planning process. A word of caution: it is vital not to mislead or exaggerate. A business plan that extols the virtues of, say, a particular skills base will lose much of its impact and persuasion if the reader finds out later that the last person to achieve this level left a year ago.

Checklist 11

Examples of people attributes:

- Their role in the organization and any particular challenges they face.
- Qualifications and experience plus any past work of an unusual but impressive nature, e.g. membership of a pioneering research team.
- Notable awards and appointments to boards, civic duties etc.
- Publications and contributions to professional bodies.

Hobbies and private interests should be avoided unless they are particularly noteworthy and link to the business, otherwise there is a danger of trivializing the message. For each person the summary should be brief and impressive. Try to avoid repeating similar phrases for different people, such as 'graduated from', 'joined us in', 'promoted to' etc. Each person's description should be individually tailored and relevant. The aim is to back up the business in a positive way while showing that all of the key people are well qualified, experienced and interesting individuals.

Checklist 12

Examples of human resource policy areas:

- Commitment to developing staff potential, both personally and for the wider benefits of patients, services and the rest of the work-force.

- Medical school/teaching hospital links.
- Requirements for minimum qualifications and acceptable professional standards.
- Training schemes and awards, such as sponsoring staff for National Vocational Qualifications (NVQs) and attainment of Investors in People awards.
- Defined links between the human resource policies and parts of the mission statement or stated objectives, as appropriate.
- Performance assessment and any related pay scales.

The balance between brevity and detail is difficult to achieve, but the right balance in this part of the plan can inspire significant goodwill from the reader.

MARKETING INFORMATION

Marketing is a key aspect of any business. In the health service it is also politically sensitive. Customers will have to be clearly identified and the products and services they demand be provided to the required standard at the best price. Who is the customer of the service? Is it the patient, the GP, the health authority or even, perhaps, the taxpayer? The effective customers for some business units will be other business units within the same organization. The products and services provided to one customer might well be questioned or challenged by another. Perhaps the provision of personnel services or management consultancy to a purchasing unit might be thought wasteful by 'taxpaying customers' or their political representatives. Those working in the health service will usually see the patients as the most important customers. Within the business planning process this will be recognized, while the relative claims of all the 'customer' groups will need to be analysed and addressed pragmatically.

Competitors will also need to be identified and the best strategy worked out for dealing with the competition. The market may lend itself to subdivision according to services, customers, geography etc. and different pricing policies and strategies may be worked out for each.

Quite often it is possible to identify a 'core' business. In the case of the health services this would be the medical, surgical, mental health etc. divisions that form the basis of current operations. The marketing of core business services will be central to the marketing strategy. At the same time, new and developing business services will need to be nurtured and marketed properly if the core is to match the changing needs of customers. It is often critically important to identify the potential of non-core activities and whether or not these have the capability to become core services in the future or will simply remain peripheral to the core business. A simple example is the distinction between, say, income from car-parking in the hospital grounds, which is clearly likely to remain peripheral, compared to a pharmacy that shows potential for expansion.

Promotional planning will be needed for different services and products to meet existing or potential markets. This is particularly so for core activities and for new products and services. The characteristics of the customers, the price the market will bear and the costs of bringing these products and services to the customer, including the costs of promotion, will need to be planned well in advance and updated if required.

Marketing is considered in detail in Chapter 6.

FINANCIAL INFORMATION

Although this book is not intended for accountants or any other profession in particular, we assume that business planners will have reasonable access to financial expertise. This does not mean that anything financial can simply be 'thrown' at the accountants. Some understanding of finance is an integral part of management, just as much as basic personnel management or appreciation of service standards. Checklist 13 sets out some of the more commonly useful types of financial information. Chapter 7 discusses this area in more detail.

Checklist 13

Broad types of financial information and their uses:

- Receipts and payments projections (cash based budgets): vital for monitoring cash flows and managing investment and borrowing. Usually combined with bank account information under the direction of a funds manager. These projections are usually vital from a corporate standpoint even if not so useful to individual business units.

- Periodic profit and loss or income and expenditure statements (accruals basis): whereas a cash basis records real money flows, an accruals basis records the income due and payments owed – vital for monitoring economic performance. Many variations of these statements can be used to measure progress towards financial targets, such as the rate of return on capital employed (profit or surplus for the year/a valuation of assets for the year).
- Capital and revenue budgets: capital refers to expenditure on basic, usually revenue-generating, assets. These include major works and repairs expected to last for over a year. Revenue budgets outline the day to day running costs and income. Budgets can be prepared on many assumptions, and it is almost as important to check these assumptions as the detail of the budget itself. Budgeting is as much an art as a science and will almost certainly require expert advice.
- Periodic management accounts: these take many forms, but all attempt to provide information for control and decision making. They are usually proactive (as opposed to the reactive published financial statements – see below). Management accounts will typically provide cost information on activities, material and labour costs, and variations between budgets and actual costs, usually with explanations. They may also include ongoing cost comparisons between, say, in-house provision and the cost of purchasing from outside suppliers. As with budgets, expert advice may assist in understanding how these accounts were compiled and can be used.
- Published financial accounts: although these are provided on a historic basis relating to the previous financial year and will usually require expert interpretation, they provide a useful opportunity to compare one organization with others. Most of the entries are standard ones prepared in established ways and lend themselves to well-established appraisal methods.

FORECASTING AND MONITORING

The hallmark of a good business plan is the selection of the information that matters for planning from among all of the other accounts, costings, sales projections and resource data that may be produced for ongoing management purposes. Information that enables progress towards meeting planned targets and objectives is crucial in this respect. Indeed, it may well be the case that some of the information for forecasting and monitoring such progress has to be generated in addition to information required for other management purposes. If this is the case to any large extent, the adequacy of existing management information or the continued relevance of the planned objectives – or both – may be called into question.

CAPITAL PROJECTS

Major capital projects usually have a profound and reciprocal impact on any business plan. It is often the business planning process for the organization as a whole that inspires the capital projects in the first place, and such projects often then become an important feature of the wider business plan. In essence, the general approach to business planning adopted in this book is suitable for dealing with capital projects and any other development. However, the National Health Service has issued specific guidance for capital projects, linking these to the Government's Private Finance Initiative and requiring a business case to be put forward for funding purposes. These issues are discussed in more detail in Chapters 8 and 9.

CONCLUDING POINTS

In this chapter we have outlined the basic elements of a business plan. The outline is not intended to be followed slavishly. The following chapters discuss some of these developments in more detail.

CASE STUDY 5   OUTLINE BUSINESS PLAN

Fitlake Mental Health Services NHS Trust

This case study shows the typical format of a business plan for a small health service Trust. It is along the lines suggested in Checklist 10 and is the outcome of the process suggested in Figure 2. The case study assumes that the supporting work on finance, marketing, human resources and the relevant operational aspects has been carried out along the lines suggested in Chapter 4 and considered in detail in later chapters. At this stage we seek to give the reader a flavour of the outcome rather than all of the detailed steps.

The Trust's plan is based on an annual cycle, in which it is reviewed every year within a longer five-year strategic business plan. This case study therefore considers the detailed position of the unit as expressed in its annual business plan.

The outline contents of the business plan are set out below:

- Foreword;
- Unit mission statement;
- Executive summary;
- Business and environment;
- Corporate framework;
- Current business unit targets;

  - Operational targets;
  - Financial targets;
  - Marketing targets;
  - Quality targets;
  - Human resources targets;
  - Capital and estates targets;

- Appendix 1: Staffing profile (not included in the Case Study);
- Appendix 2: Financial profile (not included in The Case Study).

Foreword

The Fitlake Mental Health Services NHS Trust is at the forefront of meeting patient needs both within special care facilities and within the wider community. This is achieved within the framework of the Trust's wider corporate objectives.

For the forthcoming year the most important management objective is to implement planned improvements in quality assurance and marketing, while remaining economically viable. Business targets have been set to ensure that this is achieved and provide a sound platform for success in future years.

A.T. Opper
Chief Executive

Unit mission statement

Fitlake Mental Health Services strives to maximize the quality of health care provided to all its patients.

Executive summary

The annual business plan is designed to harmonize with and fully support the corporate Five-Year Strategy. Three business object-ives are critical to the plan for this year; the first two are of strategic importance:

1. To meet our quality enhancement targets.
2. To expand our activities into work for the Crown Prosecution Service and extend the facilities for drug and alcohol abuse treatment.
3. To improve our financial performance, maintaining a balanced budget and meeting all NHS finance targets.

These and other related objectives can be achieved within the time scale of one year and will provide a sound basis for the future development of business over the medium term.

Business and environment

The Trust operates under the 1983 Mental Health Act. The gen-eral environment is one of increasing demand for the services outlined below and for increasing cooperation with voluntary organizations and local government. The geographical position of the Trust, in a mixed urban and rural setting surrounded by several health authorities, makes this an ideal setting for expanding activities into a wider range of services than are cur-rently provided.

Acute mental illness

Inpatient beds are provided at Little Bank Hospital psychiatric unit, although patients are also cared for on an outpatient basis and in conjunction with other agencies.

The long-term mentally ill

This service is provided in conjunction with Fitlake County Council Social Services Department. It aims to support the men-tally ill as close as possible to their community and home en-vironment. It also provides support for their carers.

The elderly mentally frail

A small number of inpatient beds are available at Little Pond Hospital, although most of the work is undertaken by multidisciplinary teams based at the hospital and nearby council-run homes.

Those with learning disabilities

Community-based residential care and other support services are provided in conjunction with teaching and training establishments, volunteers and council-run homes.

Drug and alcohol abuse

Services are provided in conjunction with three locally based voluntary organizations centred on a special unit at Fitlake Hospital.

Opportunities for expansion

The marketing plan identifies the potential for a second special drug and alcohol abuse facility and new work for the Crown Prosecution Service.

Corporate framework

This part of the plan summarizes the strategic approach of the Trust to the three critical business objectives outlined on page 44.

Quality

The unit is committed to providing the highest quality care totally in line with the corporate objectives, to meet the needs of patients within agreed resources. The staff of the unit have all contributed to quality awareness meetings and one of the senior consultants has taken on the role of quality liaison manager nominated to coordinate quality assurance measures throughout the Trust.

Marketing

The Trust has set up a marketing task force from its own management and clinical specialists and aided by a marketing consultant. This group has a permanent remit to improve the marketing of existing services to existing and new customers, and of new services to existing and potential customers.

Financial

The corporate financial strategy envisages an increase in funding from purchasers, primarily, that is, from Fitlake Health Authority but also from Fitlake County Council and other local agencies and voluntary groups. The immediate financial objectives for the Trust are to meet the financial targets set by the NHS Executive and to maintain a balanced budget during the planned expansion of activities for the year.

Current business unit targets

The objectives outlined in the previous section relating to the corporate framework need further disaggregation into practical short-term, i.e. one-year, targets. These have been, for convenience, classed into:

- Operational;
- Financial;
- Quality;
- Marketing;
- Human resources;
- Capital and estates.

Operational targets

There is a five-year strategic objective to reduce death rates from suicides and to reduce cases of attempted suicide. The current planned targets should be seen against this.

1. A specific 5% reduction in the death rate from suicides has been set for the current year.
2. A specific 10% reduction in the suicide death rate for the severely mentally ill has been set for the end of this year.
3. To draft a code of practice for all staff according to the main work areas:

    - psychiatric care;
    - acute and long-term mentally ill;
    - learning difficulties;

- drug and alcohol abuse;
- mentally ill offenders;
- administration and finance;
- professional conduct;
- professional development and training.

Particular chapters and sections have already been assigned to members of staff and this year's target is to produce a first draft. This code is intended to be reviewed each year in the light of the quality policy.

4. To develop a quality policy in conjunction with the Quality Assurance Manager (see quality business targets, page 48).
5. To develop detailed work procedures where the code of practice mentioned above would otherwise be overburdened by detail.

The code of practice together with the detailed work procedures and the quality policy will form the basis of a quality assurance system in line with the unit mission. The annual review will, in subsequent years, consider the feasibility of registration of the quality system to ISO 9000 (BS 5750).

6. Each patient will be provided with a care plan along the lines of the Department of Health Directives.

This and the other measures are designed to meet the Government's 'Health of the Nation' target, i.e. 'To improve significantly the health and social functioning of mentally ill people'.

Two further 'Health of the Nation' targets have been adopted for longer term, i.e. five-year, achievement:

1. To reduce the overall suicide rate by at least 15% by the year 2000, from a 1990 baseline.
2. To reduce the suicide rate of severely mentally ill people by at least 33% by the year 2000, again from a 1990 baseline.

Financial targets

The key financial business targets for the current year are:

1. To provide monthly financial and activity management information, including income and expenditure figures against

budget, by five working days after the end of each month. These reports are to provide a basis for continuing development of the effi ciency of the Trust's services.
2. To provide an annual report and accounts in accordance with best professional practice within four months of the financial year end.
3. To meet the Trust's financial targets as set by the NHS Executive.

Marketing targets

Underlying all of the marketing targets is the continuing objective of ensuring the effective operation of the marketing task force, by the unit manager. The key marketing targets for the current year are:
1. To undertake a marketing review, in consultation with Mrs S.P. Otit, the Trust's marketing consultant, to consider:
   - new products and services
   - potential new customers
   - increased marketing of existing services both to existing and new customers.
2. The demand for a second drug and alcohol abuse centre has already been identified. This will be located at Downdrain Community Hospital and work is scheduled to start later this month.
3. An expansion of the currently erratic level of psychiatric consultancy work provided towards fulfilling the statutory obligations of the Crown Prosecution Service and the Courts.
4. A further potential for expansion has been identified from services to groups and schools catering for the needs of people with severe learning disabilities.
5. To prepare an 'ideal' marketing position statement.
6. To evaluate the existing market position and compare this to the ideal position, setting a time scale for moving from the existing to the ideal position.

Quality targets

The unit has recently adopted the latest revised Patient's Charter embodied in the latest edition of the Trust's own patient's charter.
   Targets on quality attainment will be reviewed annually at the same time as in cooperation with operational targets relating to

patient care. This review will be used to update and amend the Fitlake Mental Health Care Code of Practice.

The key quality related business targets for the current year are:

1. To draft a quality policy for the unit in conjunction with all of the unit's operational management (see also operational targets, page 46).
2. To contribute to the total quality management initiative of the Trust via the quality awareness meetings and the work of the quality liaison manager.
3. To prepare a quality system manual based on the Fitlake Mental Health Care Code of Practice and detailed work procedures. It has yet to be decided whether the quality system manual will be a separate document from the Code or form a defined section within the Code.
4. To initiate a series of quality assurance audits based on a quality assurance plan.
5. To be in a position to review the quality assurance system at the end of the year with a view to setting a time scale for registration to the independent quality standard BS EN ISO 9000 or 9002, as appropriate (formerly BS 5750).

Human resources targets

The key human resources business targets for the current year are:

1. To prepare a post and skills review for all unit staff in conjunction with the Trust's personnel services unit.
2. To prepare an annual human resources budget matched to the financial budget (see page 47).
3. To prepare an up-to-date job description for each unit employee.
4. To commence a systematic job evaluation covering every employee of the unit within two years.

Capital and estates targets

The key capital and estates business targets for the current year are:
1. To prepare, as part of the Trust's property terrier, an up-to-date property portfolio covering the units' premises or share of premises.

2. To cooperate with the financial services department in preparing the annual capital investment programme and the capital income and expenditure budgets. No major capital expenditure is planned for the current year.

Summary of case study

In this case study we have focused on a small NHS Trust. The case has outlined one possible breakdown of a business plan – in this case largely geared to an annual business cycle. At this level, detailed and particular management targets must be formulated in a manner that enables meaningful assessment in output terms of what has to be done and by when.

The references to a corporate framework highlight the need for widespread cooperation and coordination at board level, an issue covered in more detail in Case Study 14 on page 107.

Key learning points

1. Business plans are made up of a wide range of related components, which must be presented in a **coordinated** manner so that the strategic objectives are clearly supported by lower order objectives and targets.
2. Behind the static appearance of the plan is a **dynamic** process that calls for regular planning on at least an annual basis.
3. **Typical components** are likely to be included in a wide range of business plans.

Chapter 5

The Mission and Strategic Objectives

MISSION STATEMENTS

Broad policy objectives will be needed to focus an organization into a defined role and give it a clear purpose. Various terms can be used for the part of the plan that sets the overriding and strategic objectives. The term 'mission statement' conveniently conveys this sense of importance, purpose and fundamental nature.

Sometimes a few, short, simple words – for example, 'we provide a prompt ambulance service to a high standard' – will suffice. Sometimes detail such as national targets, service commitments, equal opportunities etc. will need to be mentioned. What matters most is that mission statements are meaningful in relation to the organization and understood by managers, work-force, clients, customers, suppliers and anyone else who is affected by the 'mission'. It is rarely important for the precise wording of the mission statement to be remembered; few can be so short and memorable. Rather, the key message needs to be understood and spread, as the values and objectives expressed in the statement are taken on board by the whole organization. This is more inspiration and leadership than management.

The statement will clearly need to embody the objectives of the organization, either explicitly or implicitly. In the health services it is likely that the objectives will include published statements and targets, and an explicit approach is likely to be prominent. Implicitly, however, health services are bound up with moral standards, personal goals, operational influence and a host of opinions and conflicting priorities that continue to exist independently of any explicit objectives. It is essential that explicit objectives are clear at all levels of management and, as discussed above, are mutually supportive, i.e. all working towards the same mission. Managers will find it impossible to accommodate and reconcile any implicit objectives and standards to the explicit objectives of the service if the latter are not clear. If the plan fails to achieve reconciliation of objectives on paper, it is virtually certain to be ignored or bypassed in the day to day work of the managers.

The plan should allow for the honest revelation of problem areas and highlight objectives that are difficult to reconcile. Indeed, the very process of identifying such difficulties is one of the main advantages of the business planning process. Harmonizing objectives is as much an art as a science, and this is exemplified in the case studies.

Choosing the right mission statement

Examples of mission statements are given in Checklist 14; further examples are outlined in the case studies. The ones below relate to single business units within an entire health Trust, where one or two key issues such as speed of response or quality of work are critical. It is useful to compare these to the revised mission statement arrived at in Case Study 14.

Checklist 14

Example mission statements for individual units:

- We will respond swiftly and professionally to all emergency calls.
- We will provide an efficient, effective and caring recovery service to all our post-operative patients.
- All operations will provide good value for money and be completed on time to the highest professional standards.

Such statements might at first appear little more than vague generalizations, but by writing down those aspirations that encompass the core values and rationale of your business unit, direction and purpose are strengthened. The direction and values articulated in lower order management objectives and performance targets are guided towards the mission, and any wasteful or counterproductive activities become easier to spot and more difficult to justify. This becomes more apparent when one considers poor mission statements. The key rationale for the unit may have been missed, direction may be lacking or confused, and in many cases what has been achieved is no better than a 'wish list', suggesting that competing factions have all wanted their aims included. See Checklist 15, and consider the revision of mission statements presented in Case Study 14.

Checklist 15

Examples of poor mission statements:

- All operations will be carried out by fully qualified practitioners to the internally agreed standards.
- Post-operative patients will be cared for according to the agreed instructions for each case. Staff conditions and pay will be according to the ... scale, with all staff entitled to ... days training per annum. The budget will not be exceeded.
- The service will be ranked in the top quartile of performance figures published by ... Quality is paramount.

One possible approach to arriving at or reviewing mission statements is by repeatedly asking the question: can we be criticized by patients, staff, other professionals or ourselves yet still satisfy our mission?

If the answer is yes, the mission statement needs to be redrafted. In this way several drafts of the proposed mission statement will be 'fine tuned' until the final version subsumes all of the agreed purposes of the unit. At the same time this approach helps to sort out and disregard irrelevant considerations and wasteful objectives.

A more dynamic approach may be required for the mission statement of the organization as a whole, say a major Trust hospital. Often a 'brainstorming' session of the board will be helpful. Nevertheless, even for an entire organization the above question can be most useful by helping the board to focus on essential purposes.

Consider the first example from Checklist 15. It is quite conceivable that the 'agreed standards' are totally inadequate or that one of the main complaints of patients is of long delays. Clearly, these concerns would not be catered for by the stated mission. By comparison, the third example in Checklist 14 could not be satisfied if either of these, or most other possible inadequacies, were to exist. The issue of whether practitioners are suitably qualified may be of value in controlling 'inputs' but is likely to confuse rather than clarify, and says nothing about the 'outcomes' or mission that the unit wishes to achieve.

The second example from Checklist 15 shows what is essentially a collection of lower order management objectives and targets cobbled together with no attempt to give direction. Each may well be relevant to a particular target or standard to which staff are expected to conform, but the purpose of this conformity is not clear. It raises a lot of unanswered questions, such as: Will staff training result in any benefit to the individual or the service? If training is critical to the service should it be included in management objectives? Would the lack of training have much effect on the output of the unit or its customers? Does the training entitlement merely satisfy an across-the-board personnel requirement or established condition of service, or is there a continuing need for new skills? Is the training entitlement actually taken up by staff?

The third example from Checklist 15 might be appropriate if being ranked in the top quartile is synonymous with a desired mission. Unfortunately, in practice such 'competition-like' targets often become an end in themselves, even to the extent that reputations are put at stake. This type of example might well be a useful measure of particular operational performance that helps to achieve the mission but is not usually a credible mission in itself.

Deciding where you are in relation to the mission statement

Relating your current activities and position to the mission statement can involve some considerable heart-searching as well as fact finding. For many business units the financial position will be crucial: The accounts and other financial information outlined in Checklist 13 can often provide a useful starting point.

Many managers will have sunk much time and effort in presenting their part of the organization in the most favourable light possible, to both internal and external clients. It is easy to believe one's own propaganda, and usually fatal too. Business planners must be honest with themselves at this early stage of planning if the rest of the plan is to have a chance of success. The current position must be assessed honestly 'warts and all'!

Operational information, facts and statistics are no less important than financial ones. In the short run it is only on the basis of how the business unit is run and performs that the customer or patient will judge it. Particular problems such as long waiting lists for specific treatments, and poor visitor and outpatient facilities, especially signposting and reception facilities, should be noted. Successes and positive features should also be noted. For example, reputations for particular expertise or for being a nationally or internationally recognized centre for a particular treatment can be exploited to the full in any business plan.

Checklist 16 sets out some of the more likely potential sources for assessing the current position.

Checklist 16

Examples of potential information sources for assessing the current position:

- existing plans (of any type) and information showing how well these have fared;
- policy statements, existing management objectives etc;
- internal regulations and standing orders;
- treatment statistics;
- sales returns;
- occupancy rates;
- output measures (see, for example, Checklist 8);
- input measures (see, for example, Checklist 7);
- cost summaries, activity-based reports, production or service summaries etc;
- marketing initiatives;
- board minutes;
- reports to the audit committee;
- staffing details.

No particular priority is implied by the order in which these information sources are listed.

SWOT ANALYSIS

SWOT analysis is a well-established technique to focus information gathering on achieving the mission. SWOT stands for

Strengths, Weakness, Opportunities and Threats. This is where the heart-searching starts. Clear-minded objectivity is called for. It is often difficult for managers to be objective about their own organizations and their professional concerns.

Strengths	Weaknesses
Opportunities	Threats

Strengths and weaknesses can be analysed largely from looking at the organization itself and the people it has working for it. Comparisons can be made, both over time and by comparing the organisation to others, but this exercise will be largely focused inwards to analyse internal arrangements and advantages that have already been gained. Opportunities and threats, on the other hand, must be analysed largely by looking outwards to the wider economic, social, regulatory and trading environments, from local competitors to international demand for organ transplants.

Checklist 17 contains likely factors to include in a SWOT analysis. Some items will in practice appear in more than one 'box', depending upon the circumstances. For example, a particular reputation may be strength or a weakness; a new piece of legislation may offer both threats and opportunities.

Checklist 17

Examples to consider during a SWOT analysis

Strengths

- widespread popular demand for a high quality health service;
- good local reputation;
- recognized quality achievements, e.g. ISO 9000 (BS 5750);
- large population in close geographical proximity;
- no nearby competitors;
- recent capital investment;
- high building standards;
- low staff costs;
- high staff morale;
- high skill levels;
- strong links to the local community;
- strong financial position;

Weaknesses

- the reverse of the aforementioned strengths apart from the first one;
- a particular vulnerability to changes in political policy and in professional best practices;
- an increasing proportion of the population that is ageing and on declining real incomes (this could be a strength if it can be used to attract services and funding).

Opportunities

- favourable shifts in national or local government policy, particularly those giving advantage to one organization;
- technological innovations;
- identified demand for new or improved services;
- opportunities to introduce more efficient work practices;
- new population moving into the catchment area;
- new transport links that effectively expand the catchment area.

Threats

- unfavourable shifts in policy;
- technological innovations;
- work practices that are starting to become outdated;
- increasing competition from other health service providers;
- reducing demand for services via reducing population, worsening transport links etc.

All of the fact finding and searching will count for precious little if at the end of the exercise the facts and opinions do not shed light upon achieving the mission. The question that must be asked repeatedly is: how can the costs, treatment statistics, strengths, weaknesses and all the other facts and analyses be viewed in terms of our strategic objectives? In particular:

1. If the facts, costs, statistics etc. are of no relevance to the objectives why are they being produced or collected in the first place?
2. If a line of analysis sheds no light on the strengths, weaknesses, opportunities or threats, why bother continuing to pursue it?
3. If the absence of an activity has no effect upon the explicit or implied objectives of the mission, can the activity be scrapped?

PLANNED ACTIVITIES TO ACHIEVE AND MAINTAIN THE MISSION

The mission statement cannot be decided in isolation.

Fundamental objectives will probably have been known or implied from day to day work. Such existing objectives may have been consciously planned, accepted on the basis of experience and tradition, or required by law.

The earlier parts of the plan will have provided the detail of where the organization wants to be – the mission statement plus clear management objectives. Also, the earlier analysis of current activities and position in relation to the mission statement should provide the detail of where the organization is now. This part of the plan provides activities to link up the two earlier parts, showing how to get from where the organization is to where it wants to be.

All of this is easier said than done, as will become apparent. The work undertaken to consider the current position in relation to the mission statement will tend to merge naturally into this final part of the plan. Checklist 18 lists briefly some of the more common methods of getting from where the organization is now to achieving its mission.

Checklist 18

Methods to achieve and maintain the mission

- Regular and objective measurements of progress towards objectives at all levels in the organization.
- Prompt assessment of any changes required in the light of the preceding method.
- Detailed agreement on the steps expected of each key individual or group to meet management objectives and performance targets.
- Clear communication of the mission to all staff, their role in its attainment and the need for their commitment and motivation.
- Honest explanations of events, good and bad, and the reasons for management decisions or why reasons cannot be given openly.
- Identifying and scheduling planned improvements.

CONCLUDING POINTS

Without direction and clear consensus regarding basic aims, opportunities to benefit from change and to ensure that the whole organization works with a minimum of conflict will be lost. Agreeing a clear mission and strategic objectives gives this direction to an organization, enhancing leadership and management throughout.

As well as the following Case Study, Case Study 14 is particularly relevant to this chapter. It has been presented later in the book to ensure that readers have covered all of the relevant material beforehand.

CASE STUDY 6   SWOT ANALYSIS

Fitland Health Services NHS Trust Community Services Unit

The Community Services Unit within Fitland Health Services NHS Trust had received substantial additional funding as a result of government emphasis on primary care. It had attracted new people and was regarded as one of the most effective providers in the area.

The Community Services Unit had been one of the first to realize that success need not be limited to the traditional locality covered by the Fitland Trust. Clear service strategies, controlled quality of service and management competence meant that desirable services could be provided over a wide area. The two major purchasers in the area were spending more with Fitland each year, both within the Trust boundaries and in neighbouring areas.

The three individuals responsible for the success were Terence Ash, the unit director, Andrew Opper, his general manager, and Gita Bansal, the senior nurse. They had formed an effective team. Terence was the 'shaper', pushing ahead relentlessly with change. Andrew was the thinker. Ruthlessly analytical, he was constantly mentally dissecting the service, the market and the unit's achievement. Gita completed the trio beautifully, she was a natural 'people person'. She could sell Andrew's ideas to the staff, translating Terence's drive into something to which people could respond.

Perhaps surprisingly, the Community Services Unit had never produced a formal business plan before. They had their own consensus which had never been put on paper. The demand of the chief executive, Irene Alumsum, for formal planning had probably come just in time. Without clear documentation, the unit would have been prone to a number of weaknesses. Links with the Trust's acute services were becoming strained; the most successful community services were beginning to be developed without reference to the other components of the business; communication with the Trust board and senior management was about to suffer.

Terence had a natural feel for where to expand services. Gaps in the market seemed to rush out and grab his attention. Terence was also very good at talking to purchasers. He was always in contact with the two local health authorities and the GP fundholders. Because the emphasis on primary care was new, Terence realized that health authority purchasers were more than keen to work with providers to chart the way ahead. The better GP fundholders were also happy to work with the Community Services Unit to develop stronger services for their patients. So when Andrew, Terence and Gita sat down to prepare a formal business plan for the chief executive, all three were interested to see what would materialize from the process.

Terence started by commenting that the unit had developed very quickly over the past two or three years, making Irene's demand for a formal business plan timely, by allowing the team to take stock and identify the unit's strengths and successes relatively objectively while continuing its pioneering work.

Gita was concerned about whether business planning would change the direction of how the unit was developing. Terence commented:

> 'We all know the business inside out. What we need to do essentially is to brainstorm what we do, sort it out into clear issues and set straightforward objectives for us to achieve over the next few years'

In response to this, Andrew suggested that they got down on paper a clear SWOT analysis on the unit. Terence proposed that they pretend to be considering whether to make a bid to take over a neighbouring unit, which prompted Gita to wonder, 'Why the quasi-commercial scenario?' She knew that Terence loved the idea of being businesslike; because he had never worked in the private sector it had all the lure of the unknown to him. Perhaps that was in itself a weakness. Then again, perhaps it was a strength.

Starting with strengths, Gita identified the unit's greatest strength as its staff: 'They are all we could hope for'.

After about half an hour the team had prepared the following rough list of strengths, weaknesses, opportunities and threats.

Strengths
1. Motivated staff.
2. Management expertise in community care business.
3. Management committed to growth.
4. Growing market share.

Weaknesses
1. Perceived as a monopoly provider.
2. Subject to considerable change in a very short time period.
3. Possibly overambitious programme of development.
4. Limited capital to fund development.
5. Limited senior management time.

Opportunities
1. Continuation of change process and increased funding likely in future.
2. Ageing population.
3. Private Finance Initiative is opening up market for trusts to join consortia to provide care in wider area.
4. Gap in quality between 'good' and 'poor' suppliers perceived by purchasers to be widening.

Threats
1. Possible change in government policy limiting the possible range of management solutions to health-care issues. (All three managers were not up to date with political parties' health-care policies!)
2. Poor relationship with Trust senior management.

Once these lists had been produced, the discussion of their importance went on for some time. Andrew was keen that they should be able to summarize the 'mission' of the unit. To help them do this and to test the importance of the SWOT issues identified, he forced them to go through the 'So what' test. The following discussion ensued:

Terence: 'First strength, "motivated staff". So what!, What is the benefit to us of motivated staff?'
Sally: 'They do the things you want them to do quickly and well without you having to ask more than once.'
Andrew: 'OK, quality, efficiency and savings in management

time. That seems to be quite illuminating to me. I now have a clear and concise view of that strength.'

Terence: 'Third strength, "management committed to growth".'

Andrew: 'So what!'

Terence: 'So we think growth is a strength.'

Gita: 'But if I were an old person receiving district nursing care after a heavy fall would I see the unit's commitment to growth as a strength? I might see it as a weakness. I might be worried that a commitment to growth meant that senior management were more interested in their own careers than in looking after old people.'

Terence: 'But you would be wrong. We provide high quality care because we can see that ... see that a sightly bigger unit can attract higher quality staff at all grades leading to a stronger service to our patients.'

Gita: 'It seems to me that "management committed to growth" is probably a strength now but could turn into a weakness once we get beyond a certain size. Why were Trusts set up? One reason was because small is beautiful.'

The 'so what' test had been useful on this occasion. The strength was a strength but it could soon become a weakness. In addition, they had all learnt a little more about the unit and about how their own aspirations were affecting its development.

At the end of the meeting they came to the conclusion that the unit's mission was 'higher quality services through diversification and growth in the medium term'. It was not a slogan to win the hearts and minds of the public, or even of the staff. However, it did clarify some of the strategic issues affecting the unit and the direction in which they wished to move.

Key Learning Points

1. A SWOT analysis should be carried out **before objectives are clarified.**
2. SWOT analyses need to be done as **objectively** as possible.
3. SWOT analyses must cover **all of the major issues** affecting an organization and not just those subject to recent management scrutiny.
4. Often **strengths can also be weaknesses** and opportunities threats (and vice versa).
5. The '**so what**' test is a useful way of analysing the real significance of SWOT issues.
6. The SWOT analysis can lead to the formulation of a '**mission statement**'.

Chapter 6

Marketing

MARKETING IN THE HEALTH SERVICES

Marketing holds pride of place in many traditional business plans (the main rival to marketing for this position is probably financial projection). If you cannot sell what you produce all your efforts will have been wasted. In the health service the same broad considerations apply. Yet the situation of marketing is often quite different to that from which most business plans in industry and commerce are prepared.

For one thing, widespread advertising aimed at patients and those who arrange for services on their behalf is not (yet?) undertaken on the same scale as by private suppliers or the private health care sector. Advertising between actual and potential purchasers and providers is done discreetly and more in the manner of exchanging technical information and networking.

Nevertheless, marketing, even if it lacks the brashness of the private sector, is becoming increasingly important within the NHS. Information on new needs and potential services will be exchanged and reputations will be built up or tarnished. Track records, the availability of facilities and the quality of staff will be marketed actively but discreetly. Providers are nearly always trying to forge links and obtain work from an expanding range of purchasers. They wish both to expand their client base and income, and to avoid the insecurity and lack of autonomy inherent in dependency on a single main purchaser. Purchasers, too, will often prefer a 'portfolio' of providers to increase their ability to switch between them on the basis of performance and to encourage competitive efficiency.

Much of the contractor's or provider's marketing effort is concentrated into relatively short time spans as major contracts come up for renewal. Continuing renewal of numerous revenue-based purchasing arrangements is also important. Information on all aspects of the contractor's organization and the type of works undertaken, well-prepared marketing literature, annual reports, and, of course, the business plans or selected parts of these: all of this information may need to be brought to the attention of the potential client/purchaser. The marketing approach and costs will need to have been incorporated into the contractor/provider's business plan before any tendering takes place.

This marketing activity, in response to formal invitations to tender or informal requests from clients, is largely reactive. Traditional marketing strategies in the context of private sector business planning tend to be far more proactive. The fact that the vast majority of health service finance tends to come via government funds gives far less freedom to the purchaser, even within the internal market arrangements, than would be the case in a totally private sector situation. Purchasing needs and any purchasing strategies still tend to be driven by policy and by the strategies and business plans of purchasing units. There is far less probability of 'hitting upon' or developing a new demand from the supplier side or the service relationship than in many free market situations, where the market for the supplier is often made up of a relatively large number of smaller purchasers.

In the health service, therefore, the most important issue is to understand fully the needs and the wider nature of your main purchaser or purchasers. This knowledge will determine the market to which you are mainly committed. In a free market situation the suppliers, contractors and providers will often have much greater freedom over the question of, 'what market are we really in?' In the health service, unless they are based outside the service and it is essentially peripheral to their activities, the market will be very much purchaser dominated. This arises mainly from the size of the purchasers and the funding arrangements mentioned above.

Of course, this does not mean that a provider with a sound marketing strategy cannot be a step or two ahead of the purchaser's own traditional needs and other providers in the same market or locality. Certainly in the past many health service managers were content to wait until demands were placed upon them and then react. If, say, demand from local practitioners began to place strains upon ward space, finance would be sought to extend a ward. Traditional planning might have foreseen the need for additional hospital beds but this was likely to be when demand was already fairly obvious.

MARKET RESEARCH FOR MAJOR NEW PROJECTS

The building of a new hospital and similar projects will call for investment on a massive scale. This cannot be entertained without detailed research into the needs and future demand of the wider local community as well as into the full implications for funding and pricing. This more specialized aspect of market research is considered in Chapter 8.

SERVICE ANALYSIS

The SWOT analysis considered earlier lends itself not just to mission statements but also to analysis of marketing. Sometimes marketing is considered in terms of what has become called the 'marketing mix'. This generally involves analysing the opportunities available (in terms of factors such as customer requirements, product capabilities, timing of sales, cost of sales, the price the market will bear etc.) to obtain the maximum sales income. The format of the SWOT analysis can help here.

For example, the 'opportunities' box can be broken down into four areas:

New market, New service	New market, Existing service
Existing market, New service	Existing market, Existing service

Of course, for 'service' read 'product' when this is more appropriate.

Another example could relate to skills and services:

New skills, New service	New skills, Existing service
Existing skills, New service	Existing skills, Existing service

Yet another example relates to financing requirements:

New finance, New service	New finance, Existing service
Existing finance, New service	Existing finance, Existing service

And so on, relating the services currently provided or planned to come on stream to a range of influences and determining factors, such as who will be the purchasers, i.e. the market, what, if any new skills and retraining will be required and how service will be financed.

This approach is most useful for ensuring that all of the marketing options have been related to all of the influencing factors and rejecting the impractical as well as eventually selecting the most promising ones.

Greater marketing awareness will require detailed consideration of local conditions, for example:

- Are local housing associations or private developers thinking of building new homes in the area? What type of customers are they planning for? Young families? Single people? What income range?
- How are local council policies, including involvement in the wider government policy of Care in the Community, likely to develop? Where will political control lie after the next local election?
- Have new GPs been appointed and what hospital facilities are they likely to need? How have they reacted in previous appointments?

These sorts of questions can be researched in the same way as for any other market, despite the tendency for purchasers to be less free and more constricted by policy and large-scale contracts.

MARKETING AND 'DEMARKETING' HEALTH SERVICES

Various commentators have pointed to the risk that expectations arising from health service marketing may be raised only to be dashed. It is easy to appear to be a willing supplier of quality services. Critical questions for any purchaser are: Does the supplier have the capacity to respond to my demand? Will I have the funding to meet new demand?

If demand outstrips supply waiting lists will lengthen and the costs of dealing with urgent cases will increase. The likelihood of this scenario is increased by the fact that the internal market in the health service is cash limited, as part of the Government's control of public spending and the public sector borrowing requirement. Cash limits are not always set high enough to cater for potential demand, which will be virtually unlimited or very high for some services. Even when cash limits are relaxed delays will occur before this is reflected in waiting lists.

Supply is therefore not always sufficiently 'elastic' to meet rising demand. Such elasticity problems are not spread evenly over the whole country, and the effects can, for many reasons, be particularly harsh in some areas. Unfortunately, suppliers may be reluctant to admit to problems for fear of driving away potential purchasers. Purchasers will of course become disillusioned in time and seek other suppliers with spare capacity, but by then expectations will have been dashed and goodwill lost. Apart from inconvenience caused to patients, such mismatches must be minimized simply to be efficient.

In the health service, as with many other public services, the patient (pupil, claimant or other customer) is likely to rely entirely on the information of the doctor or other expert. He or she has no effective direct purchasing power. Consequently, any mismatches between supply and demand are likely to be further exaggerated in a way we would not expect with the more informed purchasing of cars, property, holidays and other consumer goods and services.

These problems have encouraged attempts to manage demand more directly at the local level. The use of the term 'demarketing' has become common in some circles to describe attempts to contain rising demand and tone down expectations. This is usually to counter the effects of past marketing efforts in the light of subsequently available resources, or the ability of suppliers to utilize resources. Cash resources in particular are critical, being linked to the numbers of patients, operations or other events used to recharge the purchaser.

There is nothing really new in this approach, but demarketing highlights the fact that hybrid situations can arise between the more traditional centralized style of government planning, which attempts to match supply and demand, and a free market, which allows supply and demand to find their own equilibrium.

CONCLUDING POINTS

All other efforts will be wasted if you are not able to reach a market for the services you provide. This is true no matter how good or desirable these services are.

CASE STUDY 7   OBJECTIVES AND RESOURCES

Fitland Health Services NHS Trust Community Services Unit

Having produced a SWOT analysis (Case Study 6), the Community Services Unit did not find it difficult to set out their high level and low level objectives. These are given below.

High Level Strategic Objectives

To ensure that:

1. Patients and clients who receive acute hospital treatment are effectively rehabilitated back into their normal life in the community.
2. The long-term ill and very old have the best possible quality of life within the community.
3. Mothers receive the best possible care, both before and after childbirth.
4. Children from birth to school age are healthy and have appropriate access to medical or social services should they require them.

Some debate occurred over defining 'the best possible' and other values implied in the objectives but all team members were fairly confident that their basic strategic aspirations had been included. From these high level objectives, low level objectives were then produced. These covered the services produced by the unit and the major management and resource areas that were responsible for the provision of services and hence the achievement of high level objectives. The following were considered:

- staff;
- buildings;
- management;
- communication.

Other possible areas would have been specialized staff groups, equipment, computers and general administration. It is important to note that although low level objectives can usually be categorized in terms of inputs, the objectives themselves need to relate to service outputs.

Low Level Objectives

Services
A whole range of explicit operational objectives for services were produced. For example:

- That all clients requiring a wheelchair receive one on the day of prescription or the day of discharge from hospital.
- That all clients requiring home visits from district nurses are visited within one hour of the scheduled time.
- That care of mothers during childbirth is monitored against a set of written standards to ensure that 95% of all standards and all 'critical' standards are attained.

Staff
1. To identify and implement optimum staff skill mixes in all areas of operation.
2. To continue to recruit only the highest quality of staff at each grade.

Management
3. To continue to develop and implement strong operating procedures to ensure that all work is of high quality directed at areas of greatest need.
4. To use every opportunity to increase contracts for services with local health authorities and GP fundholders.

Communication
5. To achieve effective working relationships with GPs and social services.

Buildings

6. To improve and maintain clinic facilities.
7. To build a new long-term illness centre using a Private Finance Initiative scheme.

Once they had all reread the objectives, Andrew commented, 'It's all very well having objectives but, (a) will our purchasers know about and will they buy the services we are offering? (b) do we have the people to implement them? and (c) are they affordable? It's quite all right to analyse our strengths, weaknesses and opportunities, and set out missions and objectives but all this is pie in the sky if we cannot sell, cannot provide and cannot afford to do them.'

Terence agreed with Andrew, but pointed out that, 'Last year purchasers knew what we did and bought, we had most of the people we needed and as a unit we generally keep to budget.'

Andrew objected that, 'This year we are trying to do more, and improve our service. I would say that of our low level objectives numbers 1, 3, 4, 5 and 6 are more than simple maintenance objectives. They all contain significant development areas. The skill mix objective requires that we change the current mix and manage that change – that involves people, believe it or not. All I am saying is that I don't think that we've really started the business planning process. From the way you talk and look, I feel that you believe we've cracked it all. I don't. I believe that 80% of business planning is matching desired objectives to the realities of market, human resources and money. For me, business planning is about identifying the equilibrium between market, human resources, money and objectives.'

Terence and Gita agreed that most of the work is in balancing the objectives with external and internal realities, but Terence stressed that the contribution of clear objectives should not be underestimated: 'Give me clear aims and the rest will follow'.

'What you mean is give me clear objectives and someone else will do the hard work to get them realized,' said Andrew. It was clear that both had valid points.

Looking at marketing, for example, they identified two objectives – objectives 4 and 6 – that have clear marketing requirements, although all have some sort of marketing needs because without a market there is no service. According to Gita, 'We need to look at our whole marketing policy and see how we should maintain it and develop it.'

Terence was beginning to see what Andrew meant by 80% of the work being in this area. And then of course there was implementation of the plan. One couldn't just write it and forget it. Then he remembered that that was much of what he was paid to do – plan and implement!

Key Learning Points

1. Objective setting is **only the start** of the business planning process.
2. Marketing, human resourses and finance are **major issues** within the business planning process.
3. Business planning requires the location of an **equilibrium** between resources (marketing, human resourses, finance) and objectives.
4. Finding this equilibrium is a **time consuming** process.

CASE STUDY 8   OBJECTIVES AND MARKETING

Fitland Health Services NHS Trust Community Services Unit

Terence, Andrew and Gita, were outlining the essentials of their marketing strategy, having agreed a draft list of their strategic and operational objectives. Their first thoughts on the unit's market are presented below.

Core market
1. Existing contracts in 'home area' with two health authorities and 53 GP fundholders.

Areas of Market Growth
2. Incremental increase of market in areas bordering home area with three health authorities, 20 identified new client GP fundholders and nine existing client GP fundholders.
3. Sale of new and additional services to social services departments: old persons' visiting service, delivery and maintenance of equipment for the physically handicapped.
4. Sale of care services to a charity specializing in help to the chronically ill living in the community.
5. Sale of management expertise and care services to a private sector consortium seeking to win Private Finance Initiative bids for 'children's resource centres' in northern England.

Summarizing, Andrew said:

> 'We need to check that all our objectives – both high and
> low level – are consistent with our marketing plan. We also
> need to be sure that the marketing plan supports the
> objectives.'

After stating that the unit's existing contracts are consistent with
the high level objectives, Terence went on to consider whether
the ideas for new markets also support the high level objectives:

> 'Looking at the areas for market growth we have identified,
> they satisfy our objectives to a basic extent. If we believe we
> do a good job the more people we deal with, the more will
> benefit!'

The following discussion ensued:

Andrew: 'Yes that is true and a useful concept, to a point. Clearly,
if we believed our service was not as good as that provided by
our competitors it would be immoral to try and take over their
services.'

Gita: 'I'm not sure that we should analyse on the basis of too
much metaphysics. Morality is best used as a longstop pre-
venting us from acting badly, not as a driver of too much policy.'

Andrew: 'Let's get down to specifics. Does, for instance, a bigger
market help us to rehabilitate patients after acute hospital treatment more effectively?' (High level objectives are set out in Case
Study 7.)

Gita: 'I can't answer that question without looking at the low level
objectives first. Our first low level objective was about improving
staff skill mixes. Does a bigger market help here? Only very
obliquely I would say.'

Terence: 'But low level objective 2 is about recruiting quality staff.
The two drivers here are probably our size and the perception
about the quality of our services. I think increased size provides
very significant benefits for satisfying this objective.'

Andrew: 'It probably does, at least for the more senior staff. I
would have thought it rather doubtful whether a good cleaner is
attracted to a big Trust as opposed to a small one.'

Gita: 'Looking at objectives 5 and 6, both of these are clearly going to benefit from a larger organization. Economies of scale will help us to improve our clinic facilities and will make us more attractive to potential PFI partners.'

Andrew: 'Let's look at this the other way round. We want a long-term illness centre. We know – sorry, *think* that our purchasers would like us to have one. We also think that the capital will be all but impossible to find from the NHS – it is desirable for them but not a number one priority. Therefore PFI is the only way forward. If that's the case then we must be attractive to the PFI brigade – and that means, among other things, strong marketing to all our potential purchasers.'

Gita: 'Yes, the marketing plan as drafted is a bit thin on *raison d'être*. We need to link it to our organizational objectives in a quite specific way. At the moment the marketing is very much linked to objective 4, which means it is about raising income rather than pursuing health-care objectives.'

Andrew: 'Marketing is essentially about market research and letting people know what services you can provide. I think we have started looking at this problem the wrong way around. First, we should do our market research, then look at our objectives, modifying them if necessary to meet real needs; lastly, we need to tell potential purchasers what we do and how well we do it.'

Gita: 'The last issue you mentioned – dissemination of information – is actually an operational objective.'

Andrew: 'We need to add it to our list of objectives, then.'

Terence: 'Let me get this clear. We have started to look at our objectives in terms of marketing. What we have failed to do is the market research.'

   By the end of the meeting a number of things had happened. First, the marketing plan had become more focused and specific to the objectives of the unit. 'Growth for growth's sake', which had been the basis of the original plan, had started to be replaced by specific 'smart' marketing ideas. In addition, the quality of business objectives had been improved. A new objective for improved children's resource centre services and a possible PFI partnership had been added because it could clearly be seen as a major aim of the unit. A marketing objective, essentially the revised marketing plan, had also been added as an operational objective.

Lastly, they all realized that they needed to do a lot more market research. It was not at all clear what purchasers wanted. The major issues affecting them were just not known.

Key Learning Points

1. **Market research** will be necessary before strategic or operational objectives can be finalized.
2. Marketing plans need to be **specific to real needs and objectives**.
3. Growth for growth's sake should be **avoided**.
4. Analysis of marketing issues may lead to **changes** both to objectives and marketing strategies.
5. The marketing plan will become an **operational objective** in itself within the business plan.

Chapter 7

Financial and human resources

THE ROLE OF FINANCE

Finance is often thought one of the most complex and difficult aspects of business planning. At the detailed level this is often so. As already mentioned, we assume that planners from a non-financial background will have access to accountants. In health service bodies diversity means that the detailed expertise of senior managers is often limited to their own specialisms, and advice may be required for financial specialisms such as budgeting, dealing with value added tax or the requirements for auditing. But this necessity must not be allowed to cloud the issues and the strategic objectives of the planning process.

In essence, the purpose of financial input to the business planning process is to ensure that financial resources are available to meet all stages of the planned activity on the way to achieving, or maintaining, the mission. Financial considerations of an incidental nature must not be allowed to dominate organization-wide planning considerations.

For example, if surpluses are allowed to accumulate an investment policy may be required to maximize the benefit from such funds at an acceptable level of risk. But funds management is not a core service activity of a health service body and the investment policy, while important, should not be allowed to influence the mission statement or over-complicate the business plan, otherwise the tail will end up wagging the dog.

Of course, lower down the organization's hierarchy a finance department's own business plan may contain a mission and management objectives designed to achieve a sound investment policy.

INFLOWS, OUTFLOWS AND BUDGETS

At the corporate level it will be necessary to consider the inflows and outflows of money over a period of time – the period of the business plan or the next financial year, for example. This information will be obtained from the budgeting and management accounting functions of the body. Clearly, failures to provide this basic information are likely to indicate a poor state of financial management. Modern management accounting has a varied bag of budgeting techniques at its disposal. The merits and uses of particular techniques, such as incremental, zero-based or activity-based budgeting, are beyond the scope of this book but certain critical information and key principles need to be appreciated. Also, at the corporate level the cash flow situation is critical. Forecasts of activities must be made and translated into income or expenditure, and variations in the actual from the planned position must be monitored and explained.

PRICING, UNIT COSTS AND CONTRIBUTIONS

Many activities result in readily defined units of output, such as hip replacements, responses to emergency calls, consultations and so on, depending on the nature of the business unit. Planning should take into account costs per unit and display the projected surpluses, losses, subsidy or contribution towards fixed costs. These projections will usually be required in total and per unit of service or goods provided, according to each planned course of action and level of activity proposed. This information will be critical for any decisions over:

- pricing policy;
- range of products and services envisaged;
- time required to achieve planned objectives.

depending upon the particular circumstances of the organization.

The non-financial manager may find the numerous variations in ways used to calculate unit costs confusing. It may be best simply to divide all of the costs of producing the units by the number produced or sold, although even here such figures are often open to dispute in practice. Sometimes the cost of producing and delivering is a better figure to use.

Often, once the initial 'fixed costs' (i.e. those unavoidable in the short term) have been covered, such as management and property costs, it may be best to recover only the additional 'variable' costs of production. In this situation the marginal cost of each extra unit can sometimes be quite low.

At the other extreme, it may be practical simply to charge whatever the market can bear – the going rate – safe in the knowledge that this will recover all of the costs that could possibly be incurred. Such a situation might imply a monopoly or near monopoly of a particular service.

It is impossible here to consider all of the potential variations on unit costing for the wide range of health services. The organization pays its management accountants for this sort of information. But the planners must be familiar with the rationale behind this accounting to judge whether the most appropriate methods have been used for the particular products and services included in the business plan. This in turn may affect particular objectives and marketing strategies set out in the plan.

In commercial situations it is important to ensure that all units of a product or service are sold at a price that at least makes a contribution exceeding their own direct costs of production and any further costs incurred in sale and delivery. That is, some contribution will be made to fixed costs. Otherwise the plan must include some form of agreed subsidy, or be able to forecast that this situation will soon be corrected.

In some parts of the health service, units of production can be difficult to define. This is true particularly where the commercial motive is less apparent, such as campaigns against unhealthy lifestyles or care of the terminally ill. We discussed this sort of problem earlier as one of the difficulties of measuring outputs (see the section on input and output measures in Chapter 3). Sometimes units of input can be used instead for costing purposes; sometimes other surrogate outputs can be identified, such as the number of campaign leaflets distributed. This problem often requires some form of cost–benefit analysis, the different approaches to which are too complex to reduce to a few meaningful paragraphs. However, as the term suggests, these methods weight the calculated costs against the benefits. In the health service these factors are often difficult to quantify for some services, such as trauma counselling or programmes linked to Care in the Community. For capital projects and services of a more readily quantifiable nature, particularly commercial services, cost–benefit analysis will usually form part of the initial business planning. This is true, for example, for capital investment planning (see Chapter 8).

VALUE ADDED AND ACTIVITY JUSTIFICATION

Such complexities of measurement and the production of cost–benefit analyses lead naturally to consideration of the 'usefulness' or value added by particular activities, rather than individual units of output.

Political or ethical dimensions are discussed elsewhere in this book (see Chapters 2 and 11) and will not now be repeated. Rather, the planner will need to consider how to agree a measure of the contribution of an activity to the total income, performance, or other aspect of the planned objectives or mission of the enterprise as a whole. For example, does the personnel department provide economies in the cost of recruitment? Does recruitment figure in any of the planned objectives?

Even at this macro level there may be some exceptions to this approach. Some legally required activities may add nothing of apparent value to the services provided. They are usually required for what is termed the wider public interest – the requirement to register with the Data Protection Registrar, for example. Such activities may at least be expected to show how they plan to minimize the cost they impose.

In summary, the financial contribution to the business planning process can be expected to contain elements such as those in Checklist 19.

Checklist 19

Vital elements of the financial input to business planning:

- Ensuring that adequate but not excessive finance is available at every stage of the plan.
- Monitoring and controlling cash flows.
- Providing forecasts and budgets for the organization and its constituent units for all significant activities.

- Providing useful explanations of variations between the budgeted and actual figures, and implications arising.
- Evaluating the costs and benefits of alternative strategies.
- Identifying the value added and costs incurred in each main activity.

HUMAN RESOURCES

Analysis of personnel issues is vital for all types of business planning: all planning will be implemented by people! Senior managers, middle managers and supervisors will be needed, as will specialists – architects, engineers, computer personnel. Operational staff of a wide range of skills will almost certainly be needed for almost any business planning objective. The business plan therefore needs to assess the quantitive and qualitive requirements for staff for each operational objective.

Senior management time

With increasing efficiency in most organizations, there is less and less slack staff time that can be used to implement development objectives or capital projects. This means that an assessment of the necessary staff input to achieve objectives is critical. In particular, all large capital schemes are hungry of senior management time. This is not surprising given that large sums are involved, often carrying high penalties to senior staff should things go wrong. Often the tendency is for senior people to take on more than they can properly achieve, even assuming they have the necessary skills. The reasons for this are many, and are set out in Checklist 20. Where in-house staff resources are short, the use of external consultants to manage a new project may be necessary.

Checklist 20

Reasons for senior management taking on excessive implementation work:

- Fear of things going wrong: *'I can't afford to let it out of my hands'*.
- Excitement at implementing a major scheme: *'That would look good on my CV'*.

- Lack of appreciation of the work involved: *'I will be able to do that by staying late two evenings a week for the next couple of months'*.

- Lack of appreciation of the skills and experience needed: *'Consultants are only human like you or me'*.

- Outrage at the charge-out rate of consultants: *'They charge a fortune for something you could easily do yourself'*.

- Concern that the Trust board will think that the senior management are not carrying out their responsibilities: *'They will think we are paid for doing nothing'*.

- Lack of appreciation of the important role an outside body can play: *'I talk to contractors and NHS purchasers every day; I don't need someone else to do it for me'*.

The important point is that there must be a proper assessment of personnel requirements, particularly for senior management. This is particularly important when preparing a business case for capital investment, when different business 'options' have to be identified involving different personnel requirements. This is discussed in more detail in Chapter 8. There is no right or wrong answer. If your staff have the skills and can manage heavy workloads there is no need to employ consultants. If the issue is in doubt look at the options available. Consultants are likely to suggest that it would be best if they did everything. Often, though, they can be used to carry out a few key tasks where perhaps there is heavy time pressure or where in-house skills are in short supply. It is important that the assessment of this is done honestly and soberly.

Design and works staff

For traditional building projects in-house NHS engineers and surveyors would be expected to do all of the design and planning work. It is now becoming more common to subcontract some of this work. For all major projects a clear assessment of the likely workload for:

1. each option for a specific project, and

2. for other projects running concurrently.

will need to be considered. The workload will need to be considered for each specialist. Pressure on design staff may be tolerable, while the quantity surveyors may be at full capacity.

Finance and accounting staff

Large projects need strong financial control to ensure that they do not overspend. At the detailed planning stage it is vital that senior accounting staff control the costings of projects. In many cases major projects that significantly overspend do so because the financial planning was defective, not because implementation costs were excessive. Clearly, during implementation financial control is also needed so that overspending can be avoided or highlighted early for remedial action to be taken. For building works much of this control will be provided by quantity surveyors and the project engineer or architect. However, ultimate financial control will usually fall upon finance departments.

Marketing staff

Large projects usually need marketing to purchasers, likely users and the general public. When setting out resource needs for different project options being considered in a business case, the human resource implications of marketing must be considered. In general, for a large project external marketing assistance will be needed.

Post-implementation issues

The human resources implications of projects once implemented need to be thought through carefully. A project option that requires much specialist or senior management time once completed may be financially viable but might cause significant organizational problems from a personnel viewpoint. Once the consultants have withdrawn their services, who will carry on where they left off? Will the estates department be large enough to cope with all the extra work resulting from a doubling of neighbourhood clinics? If the new buildings are fully used day to day spending is expected to increase by 30%. Will there be enough accounting staff to cope? More importantly, can the extra doctors and nurses required, with the right specialist skills, be recruited on time?

Another key human resources issue is the need to ensure that clear responsibility for managing benefits after the project is implemented has been concisely set down and communicated to staff. All of these issues need to be fully considered at the planning stage of a project.

CONCLUDING POINTS

It is vital to ensure that both money and people are adequate to meet each planned objective. Otherwise planning degenerates into wishful thinking.

CASE STUDY 9   FINANCE

Obstetrics and Gynaecology/Paediatrics (OGP) directorate, Oak Tree Acute NHS Trust

The OGP directorate were now beginning to pull together their business plan. They had set objectives at a strategic level and operationally. They now appreciated the structure of the planning process. They had evaluated the strengths and weaknesses of their directorate (not recorded in a case study) and some fairly lively discussion had taken place before a summary SWOT analysis had been produced.

At the meeting called today the OGP team were going to think about finance and their emerging business plan. To start the proceedings, Pravin Sengupta, the management accountant, defined the budget as representing the objectives of an organization in financial form, which means that it is a vital part of the business planning process. Michael Farr, the general manager, agreed with this, and added that two points could be made on the basis of this assessment: 'First, no money, no hospital. Second, budgets are not passive statements of likely future spending. They are real plans in themselves'.

Expanding on the second point at the request of Conrad Campbell, the clinical director, Michael explained, 'The overall budget we receive represents our purchasers' objectives of obtaining health care. Our plan is to further the objectives we have identified using the money we expect to receive. We need to start by identifying our likely funding for next year. Until we know what quantum of money we have at our disposal it is almost impossible to put in place firm plans.'

The finance director's lastest briefing on resources had suggested little change from last year, although specific funding for an extra paediatrician had been agreed.

The participants then went on to consider the calculation of next year's figures, on the basis of information supplied by Pravin.

	£ 000
Total budget 199x/9y	4756
Less: Funding for non-recurrent items falling out next year	(134)
Add: Full year cost of items introduced part way through 199x/9y	58
Add: Budget increases already agreed for 199y/9z	
– additional paediatrician	60
– midwifery training moneys	17
Base budget 199y/9z	4757

Pravin, giving some explanation of his figures, said, 'The budget for this year is the current budget we hold. For next year we must subtract any funding we received this year which we know we will not obtain next year. For this reason I have deducted the 'waiting list moneys which were recently agreed.' Conrad queried the reason for this, arguing that, 'If purchasers have the money this year they are almost certain to give us some extra next year.'
Pravin explained,

'By definition a waiting list initiative is only for one year. We are trying to calculate a base budget for 199y/9z so we need to exclude amounts which we know are for one year only. In that way we produce a budget of "recurrent income".'

'So we take it out because by definition it is for one year. Can we add some in for next year – we are bound to get something, aren't we?' Conrad asked. Pravin agreed:

'What we add in will be on top of our base recurrent budget. We have not got that far yet. Once we have taken out the waiting list money and one or two other small non-recurrent amounts we need to add in budget for items that are recurrent but for which funding was obtained only part way through this year. The extra money we got from the medical dean for junior doctors was from July. Next year we will get 12 months worth rather than the 9 months we will get in 199x/9y.' Lastly, I have added in the development funding we have already agreed with purchasers for next year – the extra paediatrician and the midwifery training moneys. If we know the money will be available then we should take it into account. And that gives us our base budget for next year as we perceive it now in September of the year before.'

Conrad commented, 'We had better get some funding to replace the waiting list funds that you have excluded.' Michael replied, 'Let's not think about that until we start looking at our waiting list objectives. The waiting list money is an important issue but it is only one of our many objectives. We need to look at objectives next and then start to match money to them.' Cherry pointed out that it would probably be possible to earn additional income from some GP fundholding practices, and that this ought to be added to the budget. Michael agreed that this, too, should be an objective.

When Norman suggested adjusting the figures to take account of inflation, Pravin replied:

'No, we do not need to think about inflation at this stage in the process. First, we do not know by how much purchasers will increase prices next year. Second, adding inflation really only serves to complicate at this stage. Income and expenditure will normally both be increased by inflation so it is normally best practice only to add it in once budgets are set. That means that we can ignore it for at least six months.'

Key Learning Points

1. The **budget** represents the **objectives** of an organization in **financial form**. It is not simply a passive forecast of likely future spending.

2. A major element of business planning is to **further the organ-ization's objectives** using the **funding available**.
3. *Before* objectives can be implemented the **total amount of money** likely to be available needs to be **identified** in detail.
4. Clarity of thought is required when identifying likely future budget levels. Similar funding to last year may mean a sub-stantial change in budgets once non-recurring and additional items have been taken into account. **The involvement of an accountant is essential**.
5. **Objectives** will need to be constantly **reviewed** as the busi-ness planning process continues and issues become clearer.
6. **Ignore inflation** when starting to look at budgets; this can be included once all the figures are agreed.

CASE STUDY 10   FINANCE CONTINUED (1)

Obstetrics and Gynaecology/Paediatrics (OGP) Directorate, Oak Tree Acute NHS Trust

Having identified the level of likely funding available for the busi-ness planning period, the OGP team are now starting to compare their low level objectives with the total budget they have prepared. Michael has just handed round a list of the low level objectives for Obstetrics and Gynaecology. They are similar to those discussed in Case Study 3 but have been developed further as a result of the SWOT analysis work refered to in Case Study 8.

Low level objectives

1. To treat 3% more patients than in the current year for the same total cost while increasing the quality of work.
2. To commence a research project trialing new methods of mini-mizing the extent of surgery.
3. To cut infection rates after surgery by 20% in the next 12 months.
4. To set up and implement detailed training programmes for all staff to develop their skills and flexibility and improve both the efficiency and the quality of patient care.
5. To cut waiting lists to a maximum of nine months by the end of the year.

6. To review staffing structures in wards and midwifery to increase effectiveness without increasing overall costs.
7. To monitor and analyse the number and nature of abnormalities in babies born in order to limit those cases that are preventable.
8. To ensure that league table results are on average one star better than the previous year.

They all reread the objectives they had decided upon for Obstetrics and Gynaecology at the previous meeting. They were certainly better than their first attempt a couple of weeks ago. Michael explained that they would need to go through the list of objectives, stating what tasks needed to be done. The objectives represent aspirations rather than specific tasks; the tasks now need to be isolated. Once the tasks had been identified, they could be costed, then the team could decide whether they were affordable under the projected budget. Michael emphasized the point that the objectives, in one form or another, cover all that is done within the department, which is important because the budget clearly must cover all the work of the department. Hence, if the objectives do not cover all that is done they are either incomplete or something is being done that could be scrapped.

Conrad commented that setting down all of the activities associated with each objective would be an enormous task. Michael replied:

'It is if you do literally all of them. When you do that it is known as zero-based budgeting or ZBB. If the organization is simple or you have a lot of time available then this is appropriate. For our purposes I suggest we ZBB only selected areas. I expect that improved staff structures are one area where we will analyse activities against objectives in some detail.'

As an example, the team discussed objective 7, relating to monitoring abnormalities in babies. Conrad said:

'To achieve the objective we need to record key details of the mothers' care and treatment during pregnancy and birth. We will need a database, someone to man it, and expertise to make sense of the data we collect. How much will all that cost?'

As the unit delivers about 500 babies a year, collecting the necessary data would be an onerous task. However, Cherry pointed out that much of the data would be available on the HISS module (a computerized hospital information system, which records everything that happens to a patient while in the care of the hospital), so only data validation and review before analysis would be needed. Taking this information into account, Conrad suggested that a Grade F nurse could do most of the work on one day a week, supported by a consultant and a computer person. A computer and printer with spreadsheet and database programs would also be needed. The team agreed that an existing member of staff, Jenny Hall, could do the work, but that a Grade E nurse would have to be employed for one day a week as cover. Summarizing, Cherry said:

> 'So as far as I can see, it will cost us 20% of an E grade nurse at agency rates (although an F grade will be doing the work!) and a PC with appropriate software. Presumably consultants would be able to provide the time out of their existing contracts.'

Pravin costed the proposal as follows:

Cost of implementing monitoring programme on abnormal births

	£
Agency Grade E nurse 20% whole time equivalent (WTE)	3000
Consumable stocks (say £500)	500
Annual cost	3500
Computer and software	2500
Total first year cost	6000

Norman commented:

> 'That is all very straightforward, but our budget is only £1000 higher than last year and I have got £60 000 for my extra paediatrician. Where is the money for this going to come from?'

No one could answer this question. The team decided to cost all of their objectives before becoming too despondent. Cherry had done some work with Pravin and the ward nurse managers on objective 6, relating to staffing structures.

She produced the following figures for Fisher Ward:

	Existing		Proposed	
	WTE	£000	WTE	£000
Ward manager	1	27	1	27
Grade F	2	44	1	22
Grade E	5	100	3	60
Grade D	4	66	6	99
Nurse assistants	6	72	7	84
	18	309	18	292

This change could be achieved only through skill development in three areas of nursing work. Courses are available that could teach the skills needed. For the three staff involved the training would cost £1500. But this proposal would result in a saving of £15 500 (309k – 292k – 1.5k). Cherry considered that similar savings would be available in the maternity ward but that these could not be achieved in one year. Nevertheless, the savings resulting from her proposed changes would be sufficient to enable objective 7 to be put into effect.

Key Learning Points

1. Specific tasks that will **fulfil** low level objectives need to be identified.
2. Tasks fulfilling objectives need to be **specific** so that they can be costed.
3. **Budgets** should be built up from '**scratch**' or a **zero base** where this is possible. Detailed budgeting should be used where workloads permit and benefits are likely to be greatest.
4. Objectives should cover the **entire activities** of the organization in the same way as the budget does.

CASE STUDY 11   FINANCE CONTINUED (2)

Obstetrics and Gynaecology/Paediatrics (OGP) Directorate, Oak Tree Acute NHS Trust

After the meeting discussing objectives and their financing, Pravin started to pull together the numbers they had discussed. First, he set out the detail behind the summary total budget given in Case Study 9. In this way the effect of the deduction of non-recurrent money as well as the addition of the new developments could be seen clearly by budget holders.

Having analysed the base budget for the year, he then produced another spreadsheet showing the effect on each budget line of implementing the low level objectives for the year. Where necessary, he produced detailed working papers supporting the figures shown on the spreadsheet.

Having done all this work, he discovered that the cost of implementing the objectives was £6876 above the expected total budget for the year. At the next business planning meeting, this issue was discussed first. Several suggestions were put forward: cheaper ways of achieving the same objectives could be looked for, some of the objectives could be cut or modified, or other objectives that would save money or raise net income could be added. At this point, Cherry mentioned the possibility of earning more money from GP fundholders, referred to in Case Study 9. GP fundholder income over the previous two years had been increasing steadily in the OGP directorate, faster than in the Trust as a whole. Some of those present saw this as the answer to their problems. Pravin, however, advised caution:

'We can really only include in our budget an income figure agreed with the director of finance. The issue is one of prudence. If we set expenditure budgets at an unrealistically high level because we were banking on substantial income growth then there could be problems for the Trust as a whole if we were in fact over-optimistic. All we need to do is make a strong case. If we can, then there is our income. If we can't, then how certain are we anyway? That's one way of looking at it. Second, extra income is not all ours for the taking. The price charged for a procedure must pay for all the costs of the work. About 40% of costs are outside OGP – for instance, in theatres, pathology and support services.'

After considering income from GP fundholders, the team then reviewed some of the other objectives and made small amendments to the way they were to be achieved, and hence how much they might cost. By the end of the meeting they had a plan that met strategic and operational objectives *and* was affordable.

Key Learning Points

1. Costings need to be **detailed**.
2. Budgets need to be set **prudently**, using low figures for uncertain income while providing more generously for costs to cover uncertain or contingent expenses.
3. Costings need to be at a level so that junior and middle managers can see the **effect on their departments**.
4. Once costings have been prepared it is normally necessary to **revisit** budgets to achieve objectives in a way that ensures that total costs are likely to be within budget.
5. Sometimes **objectives** themselves will need to be **revised** if they are not affordable in their original form.

CASE STUDY 12   OBJECTIVES AND HUMAN RESOURCES

Fitland Health Services NHS Trust Community Services Unit

In the haste to reform the management of the Community Services Unit after the achievement of Trust status for Fitland, Terence, Andrew and Gita had never produced a coherent human resources (HR) policy. A major theme for them throughout the business planning procedure had been managing growth. Since their growth would be based on people, they now considered it an ideal time to look at the HR implications of objectives and implementation options. On the basis of this, an HR policy, could be drawn up.

According to Terence, 'We have just drawn breath, so to speak, from the first stage of knocking this unit into some sort of shape. Consolidation would be a reasonable goal rather than more experimentation.'

They considered this aim in the light of the agreed business plan. Looking at the personnel implications of what they had been setting themselves, they realized that they would not be able to do everything at once. Gita suggested staggering the work:

'If we started on the children's centre first we could use the experience usefully for the long-term illness project.'

Terence raised some other issues:

'Then there is all the skill mix work we want to do. That has enormous HR implications. What about the use of agency staff? We will need a policy that will then have to be managed. What about appropriate training policies to buttress the new skill mixes we achieve? We will need strong policies and implementation there, too. Do we have the middle management to see all this through?'

Although they all agreed that the answer to this question was probably 'yes', Terence remarked, 'It would be very nice to see that demonstrated on paper – we need a human resources strategy.'

Andrew concluded:

'We need to tackle our human resources planning thoroughly. We have done quite a lot of planning and it does not seem unreasonable to buttress that with a human resources strategy with evidence of its achievability. We are not a small business; we have 350 staff.'

Key Learning Points

1. Health care is a **people-based business**. HR planning is therefore vital to match skills and availability of staff to the tasks in the plan. In this way business planning objectives are more likely to be achieved.
2. HR planning should cover the **long** term, the **medium** term and the **short** term.
3. Planning should cover both **service-providing** staff and **management**.
4. Plans should address **specific** business planning objectives.
5. High level business planning objectives will be addressed by analysing **strategic staffing requirements**.

Chapter 8

Capital investment planning

THE ROLE OF FINANCE

So far we have looked at business planning and its different components or stages in the context of a complete organization or department. We have also looked at business planning in a wider context than that required to meet NHS Executive requirements. However, because the capital financing requirements for NHS bodies are rather specialized, this chapter concentrates on the subject.

In the NHS there is guidance covering a range of planning documentation. Such planning will often be helpful when drawing up the organizational business plan. Conversely, the business plan may drive the more detailed planning.

CAPITAL PLANNING

Capital investment is a major area, which is usually analysed in greater depth than in the main business plan. Any organization that uses buildings and machinery will need to ensure that these are adequate and consistent with its other plans. As an example, a Trust cannot decide to obtain the funding for 50% more surgery cases unless it has the theatre capacity for this work. If it has not, then the business plan must address the investment in more hospital space. The planning for a major project, while it may be mentioned, should not normally be detailed within the business plan itself. Rather, a capital 'business case' will be prepared.

Every year the health service will typically spend about 6.5% of its total spending on capital. For the average Trust, this will mean that between £2 and £5 million will be spent annually on many medium and small projects. Even at this level, spending is substantial. However, health service organizations will periodically spend much larger sums. This will occur when a new hospital or clinic is built. When between £1 million and £100 million is to be invested in a single project it becomes clear that effective business planning procedures are needed. In the NHS much of the business planning procedure for capital is referred to as 'a business case'.

THE BUSINESS CASE

Capital investment should only be made when it is clear that such spending will efficiently further the objectives of the organization. First, then, the business case has to identify clearly the objectives that capital spending will satisfy. For example, when purchasing a major information technology (IT) system that will enhance patient data, it is important to show that it will advance quality of care and efficiency objectives. The second major task of the business case is to identify a viable option and demonstrate that it provides the best balance between costs and benefits. If three computer systems were available for the enhancement of patient data then the business case must identify the abilities of each system and their costs before demonstrating which would provide the best value for money.

Business cases carry out other tasks. They document thought processes, provide accountability and analyse risk. These and other issues are considered below. Their major functions, though, are ensuring that capital projects meet real needs and that this is done as efficiently as is reasonably possible.

We can define a capital business case as follows:

> A business case sets out the **strategic** and **operational objectives** which capital spending must satisfy, and identifies a **viable option**, demonstrating that it provides the best balance between **costs, benefits and risk**.

CURRENT ISSUES

There is nothing new in the idea of rational planning for expensive projects. However, in the modern health service business cases are topical for the reasons set out in Checklist 21.

Checklist 21

Reasons for current interest in business cases:

- The inadequacy of planning in the past.
- Trust status has substantiallly increased accountability.
- Complex and large IT projects have focused the need for detailed planning.
- The Private Finance Initiative (PFI) necessitates planning for deals to be viable.
- Shortage of public money means that the best planned projects usually have the best chance of funding.

Considering in turn each of the factors mentioned in Checklist 21, a major reason for the current emphasis on business cases is that capital planning in the past has often been carried out haphazardly. Analysis and documentation of the reasons for spending millions of pounds have been poor. Decision making has not been rigorous; both the NHS Executive and the Treasury now admit that a more structured approach to spending on major capital projects has increased the quality of decision making.

Secondly, the advent of Trusts has increased the accountability of senior management to the NHS Executive, Trust boards and non-executive directors, who are strongly averse to supporting capital projects that might fail. A clear and concise business case setting out the need for a project and a clear analysis of the options and their costs means that boards will be more likely to give approval. Accountability also means that senior managers will wish to demonstrate that their decisions were rational, if only as a protection against things going wrong later.

To some readers the current NHS structures may still appear to have weak accountability. It is fair to point out that accountability to central government has increased when compared to the lack of accountability inherent in the old system, which did not separate health planning and purchasing from health provision. However, the current system is arguably a less accountable structure than a locally financed service answerable to a local electorate.

There have been a number of disastrous IT projects in the NHS in the recent past. The well known failure of the London Ambulance Service computer and other high profile computer scandals in the early 1990s showed the need for much stronger control over IT projects. A key area for stronger procedures was at the planning process.

Since 1992 there has been a push towards involving the private sector in capital projects – the PFI. The details of PFI are set out in Chapter 9. However, the involvement of private sector partners in major projects obviously necessitates clear planning and decision making processes. Profit-making businesses have considerable incentives to ensure that any investments made are successful. Strong business cases are important to reassure PFI partners, including their bankers and shareholders, that the investment is wise.

Finally, the shortage of public funds compared to the ever rising number of possible uses brings more pressure on governments and their bureaucrats to ensure that where money is committed the project is efficient and useful. Projects that have compelling business cases will stand a better chance of funding than those without. Hence, the NHS Executive regularly publishes guidance on capital business case preparation.

RELATIONSHIP OF BUSINESS CASES TO THE BUSINESS PLAN

A Trust will normally have a Trust business plan supported by departmental business plans. In a similar way, the Trust business plan will also incorporate the business cases for significant capital projects. This relationship is illustrated in Figure 3.

NHS GUIDANCE AND CONTROL ARRANGEMENTS

At the time of writing all projects over £1 million must be approved by the NHS Executive in Leeds and all projects over £5 million by the Treasury as well (these amounts are subject to change). Clearly, planning documentation should be prepared in such a way as to satisfy their needs as well as internal requirements.

Capital finance arrangements

When the NHS spends about twenty times more on the day to day care of patients than on new buildings, equipment and computers, it is perhaps difficult to see why the NHS Executive controls the

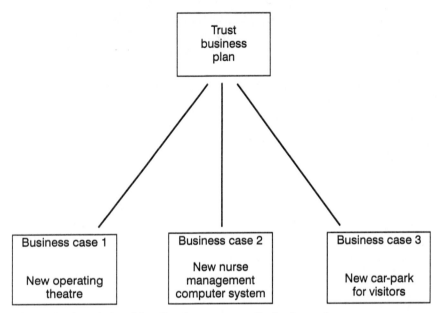

Figure 3 The relationship of business cases to the business plan

capital spending process so closely. Capital spending is, however, costly (about £2 billion is spent each year) and is a major determinant of future revenue expenditure on running the new capital schemes. It is also politically sensitive. For these reasons, the NHS Executive and the Treasury both approve all major NHS capital spending schemes at the business case stage. But there is another reason, linked to clear control of economic policy, why these two central bodies become involved.

Day to day revenue spending on patient care is clearly devolved to purchasers and thence to provider Trusts. The role of the NHS Executive and the Treasury is therefore indirect. Capital is not so fully delegated. Spending is controlled through the requirement for specific approval and the External Financing Limit (EFL). The EFL is the 'tool' that the Treasury uses to control cash spending in the NHS.

Specific capital approval

The day in, day out capital programme of small and medium projects is agreed with the NHS regional outpost each year. This covers all works and purchases up to a limit that fluctuates. For a medium sized Trust this might cover works and equipment totalling £2 million. Above this limit, all projects must be agreed by the regional outpost on an individual basis. The financial limits and authorization procedures in force at any one time will need to be checked.

Substantial projects must be agreed by the regional outpost and the NHS Executive in Leeds. PFI projects and the largest publicly funded works require specific Treasury agreement as well. To get a project past all these people, the quality of the business plan needs to be high.

Looked at as a series of bureaucratic hurdles, the process appears unbusinesslike. However, in any organization whenever large capital sums are to be spent similar hurdles usually need to be cleared. A company will have to raise cash either from a bank or shareholders. Clear, compelling business case documentation will be required. Indeed, the business planning process is very much a private sector tool for raising finance. For these reasons NHS employees or advisers may find it helpful to view the approval process in its wider perspective.

External Financing Limit

Each year NHS bodies are given an EFL figure to achieve by the NHS Executive. This is effectively a cash limit. A major component of the EFL or cash limit is the cost of the capital spending programme for the year. If a Trust wishes, say, to build a new hospital and keep to its EFL it must have obtained NHS Executive and Treasury approval for the spending so that a sanctioned EFL figure can be met.

In practice, the Treasury lends the capital finance to the Trust or other NHS body. Finance directors could theoretically find the necessary finance without borrowing from central government but no NHS director of finance would set out to breach the EFL.

NHS Executive approval is therefore required for all large capital projects. On the basis of this approval the EFL will be set appropriately. Capital spending must therefore be well planned in accordance with NHS Executive guidance. In addition to all this, Trusts must also attempt to obtain private finance under the PFI. This additional hurdle is discussed later.

CAPITAL INVESTMENT MANUAL

The latest NHS *Capital Investment Manual* was published in 1994.

This sets out best practice in the following areas:

- Project organization;
- Business case preparation;
- Private Finance Initiative;
- Managing information management and technology (IM&T) projects;
- Managing construction projects;
- Commissioning a health care facility;
- Post-project evaluation.

By following this guidance bodies will meet current NHS Executive requirements.

In this book we are mainly concerned with the business planning elements of capital spending. Readers are advised to study these areas of the manual themselves, but the following seven aspects are of particular relevance to the wider issues of business planning:

1. Three phases of NHS business cases
2. Cost–benefit analyses
3. Human resources
4. Marketing
5. Risk analysis
6. Selecting the preferred option
7. Post-project evaluation

These aspects are considered in the following subsections.

Phases of the business case

The *Capital Investment Manual* sets out three phases in drawing up a capital business case. This structure is shown in Figure 4.

Phase 1 provides the link with the business plan of the whole Trust. In this part of the business case the strategic aims of the trust are described as a basis for setting objectives for the capital scheme. This is a crucial area because capital should be spent only if it furthers the aims of the Trust.

Phase 2 involves the preparation of a planning document. Described as 'outline', the NHS Executive in fact expects about 30–40 pages. This document will require approval before funding and authorization to proceed will be given. Even if a PFI solution involving no public money or EFL adjustment were found by a

Phase 1

Phase 2

Phase 3

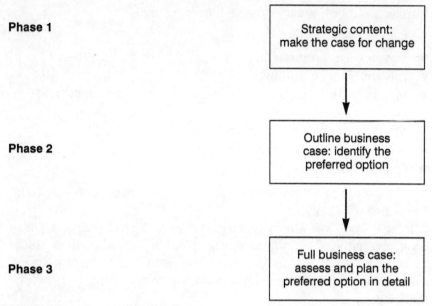

Figure 4 Preparation in three phases

Trust, approval would still be required.

Phase 3 is almost an implementation plan. Having made the decision on the preferred option, the full business case reviews phases 1 and 2, obtains formal board endorsement and plans project implementation, control and post-project evaluation. Phase 3 is not really part of the business planning process, but is the first step towards project management. For this reason we do not consider this phase in detail.

Strategic context: phase 1

The *Capital Investment Manual* calls for rigorous analysis of the Trust's 'strategic context'. This work is in essence a SWOT analysis and formulation of high level objectives. For organizations with a weak Trust business plan, the emphasis is on carrying out most of the initial aspects of the business planning process before major capital spending is sanctioned. Those Trusts with strong business plans will not have to repeat this work.

The manual sets out a series of strategic context issues similar to those raised in Chapter 5:

Where are we now?
- appraise current health-care services;
- describe the assets of the trust;
- assess financial situation and current cost structure.

Assessing demand
- the role of purchasers;
- understanding the demand for health-care services;
- competitors;
- competitive analysis.

Where do we want to be?
- understanding future needs and demands;
- assessing the scope for improvement;
- matching capital assets to service needs;
- establishing the case for change;
- affordability;
- joint proposals with universities (for teaching hospitals);
- planning the next step.

The strategic context is clearly a vital part of the business case. For the well-run organization this work should never need to be done as part of a capital business case because the organization's main business plan should have covered these issues. However, with the advent of PFI, best practice is moving towards preliminary business case documentation composed of longer, more detailed discussion of the strategic issues that a major capital project would affect. In this situation a full outline business case might be left until links with possible PFI partners had been made. This issue is discussed further in Chapter 9.

Outline business case: phase 2

This stage involves the main business planning techniques – already set out in earlier chapters – of setting low level or operational objectives, considering ways in which to achieve them and then ensuring that they can be afforded. The marketing issue is crucial where large increases in health-care capacity are envisaged. The strategic context part of the work will already have looked at this issue but usually not for each individual project. Human resources will need to be considered in detail in any capital project. The *Capital Investment Manual* is perhaps a little thin on marketing and human resources, concentrating mainly on cost–benefit analysis.

Cost–benefit analysis

Low level objectives

Organizations with clear objectives normally find these objectives relatively easy to implement. For this reason, clarity over essential issues is vital when trying to agree low level objectives. It is important to think in terms of 'outputs' or 'outcomes' rather than specific objects or 'things'. With the advent of PFI this type of thinking becomes even more important. This is because a major benefit of PFI is that the private sector contractor turns the objectives into a viable project that may satisfy more objectives than simply those of the Trust.

The risk of narrow non-outcome-based objectives is that they cover the need too thoroughly in some areas and not thoroughly enough in others. Time spent considering the essence of what is needed by defining outcomes will be well spent.

Benefits

A corollary of setting strong objectives is that they will produce outcomes that will give clear benefits to the organization. These benefits can then be measured.

Some benefits will have clear financial implications; others will have measurable benefits that are difficult to quantify financially. A reduction in missed or late appointments falls into this category. Lastly, there may be unquantifiable benefits. Increased satisfaction of patients might be thought to fall into that category. However, it is normally possible to measure benefits, and a patient/visitor satisfaction survey could be used to monitor the achievement of this benefit.

Options and benefit evaluation

Once objectives have been considered and the benefits they should provide for the organization have been identified, practical options that will satisfy these objectives will need to be worked out.

In the field of capital works, options will normally involve discussing ideas with third party specialists. For example, when considering hospital access, architects will be needed to devise improved use of space, to position lifts or escalators and to design signage. Options could be found by talking to the in-house design team, by presentations from bidding firms of architects or even through a design competition. Much would depend on the circumstances and the size of the scheme. For computer projects discussions with software suppliers will normally provide the options.

Not all of the options will provide all of the benefits. It is important that for each possible solution the benefits are clearly assessed and recorded. For computer projects in particular the various solutions will all have pros and cons.

Having identified benefits under the NHS technique these must be weighted and scored. The benefit of reception staff time reduced by 50% might be £25 000. This is clearly a greater benefit than a 5% cut in portering costs, worth only £17 000. Subjectively, though, an expected cut in outpatient appointments missed might be worth more than either of the other benefits considered. The benefits can be weighted and scored on any reasonable basis, but a scale of 1 to 10 is easy to use. Details of weighting and scoring techniques are given in the *Capital Investment Manual*.

'Do nothing' option

An important benchmark for all analysis of capital spending is the 'do nothing' or 'do minimum' option. This option will have benefits, risks and costs, just like all the others. No NHS capital business case will succeed in obtaining funding unless this option is considered fully.

Costs

The NHS technique puts much emphasis on cost analysis. The *Capital Investment Manual* works on the following principles:

- All costs must be compared to the cost of the 'do nothing' option.
- Costs must be considered on a 'whole life basis'.
- Costs must be shown as a 'net present value' (NPV) using (currently) 6% discount factors.
- Inflation is ignored.

Perhaps the most important of these points is the requirement to look at 'whole life' figures. This means that costs include all of the six categories set out in Checklist 22.

Checklist 22

'Whole life' costs of a project:

- initial capital outlay;
- annual maintenance and running costs;
- associated staffing costs;
- any income generated during use;
- estimated value of the *use* of any existing assets owned by the Trust (opportunity costs);
- residual value at the end of its useful life.

Costing must be done for each of the options identified. The timing of costs needs to be taken into account so that discount factors can be applied to achieve NPVs for each alternative. Normally service managers (that is, non-financial managers) should identify as many of the costs and income flows as possible. It is important that an accountant becomes involved at this stage to analyse all of the options and calculate the NPVs. Options with the lowest NPV are the cheapest. The practice of calculating discounted cash flows is relatively simple. However, since it is always best practice to have all costings reviewed by an accountant it is usually best to get the finance person involved at this stage.

The *Capital Investment Manual* shows in detail how costings should be prepared.

Human resources

As with all other business planning techniques, the analysis of personnel issues is vital for all capital schemes. Oddly, the NHS *Capital Investment Manual* does not dwell heavily on this issue, even though it is strongly implied when considering staffing costs for projects. Many of the human resources issues that need to be looked at were considered in Chapter 7.

Marketing

For any project it is important to know that there is a market for the outputs it will provide. A new day centre for the mentally handicapped will be useful to a Trust that has an increasing demand from purchasers for such facilities. It will be a substantial liability to a trust with falling requirements for services to the mentally ill.

An example of investment in assets where there was no demand for the outputs is given by the British Steel Corporation. In the 1970s under Sir Monty Finiston it was believed that demand for steel would continue to increase as it had in the 1960s. New and expanded plants were built to produce the extra steel. In fact, steel needs started to fall as the post-industrial society began to evolve and services started to take over from manufacturing.

Health service bodies must be careful to test the market for their 'products' by analysing trends locally and talking to key purchasers. Competitor capacity will also need to be analysed carefully. For example, Trusts near big population centres will often find it difficult to specialize in rarer conditions. Although, theoretically, there is a demand, often this will be met by competitors in a large city.

Marketing was tackled in detail in Chapter 6. The main issue to bear in mind is that although demand for a service may be strong from patients on a nationwide basis, it may be very weak locally as a priority from purchasers. Perhaps the best view to take is a sceptical one. Invest only where there is clear, unambiguous evidence of a market! Trusts are now required to obtain written support from major purchasers for large capital projects.

Risk analysis

At this stage the business case will have produced a range of costed options giving a range of benefits that will satisfy the objectives to a greater or lesser extent. The implications of each option in terms of finance, human resources and marketing will have been considered and the strengths and weaknesses of each analysed and recorded. At this stage the best option in current circumstances could be identified. However, before a decision is taken a risk analysis must be carried out.

Risk analysis of project options considers the likelihood and consequences of changes in the basic circumstances surrounding options. It is a useful technique whenever planning is carried out. The best option may be the best only in a single, perhaps ideal, set of circumstances.

The *Capital Investment Manual* outlines some ways in which risk analysis can be done. Essentially, the technique involves rescoring option benefits assuming changed in scenarios. In a hospital expansion project, for example, the plans for the largest extension would probably be higher risk than a smaller project, on the grounds that it would be less easy to guarantee sufficient patients.

Risk or sensitivity analysis is carried out numerically using weightings. It cannot be done effectively merely by discussing possible problems, although this approach will be useful in identifying risks, if not in quantifying their effects. Analyses can be done on spreadsheets, which allow for the effects of extreme risks to be modelled easily. Copies of the risk analyses will be required in the outline business case. Best practice requires that copies of the documentation should be kept so that the planning process can be reviewed before final decisions are taken. They should also be filed for future reference.

Selecting the preferred option

Once the risk analysis is complete the preferred option will become apparent. The written numerical analysis of costs, benefits and risks notwithstanding, the final decision will often involve an element of 'gut feeling'. Often different parties involved in the planning work will have different views on which option to select. A significant element of discussion may be part of the final decision making process as the major issues affecting the project are teased out.

All of the above discussion is of management processes – objective setting, benefit analysis, costings etc. These processes need to be written to achieve the quality and communication required for high quality business planning. As a separate issue, to obtain NHS Executive approval, all of the above must be recorded persuasively in a report. This is the outline business case document.

Post-project implementation

In this chapter we have looked at the need for business planning techniques to be applied to large capital projects in the light of the NHS *Capital Investment Manual*. Post-project implementation is one other major issue that should be considered.

It is easy to believe that benefits will flow from capital work. But this is far from guaranteed. A new HISS computer system in a hospital does not automatically mean that patient care will improve. Even a new hospital provides no certainty of a healthier population. Benefits have to be managed once the new fixed assets are in place.

IM&T projects and new medical equipment

Nowhere is management of benefits of more concern than with computers. Information technology is easy to buy but very much more difficult to utilize in the achievement of operational objectives.

The reasons for this are not difficult to find. Computers primarily produce data. Data by itself has little direct use; it is *information* that is useful. Ensuring that information is obtained from computer data is often not easy. Ensuring that information is obtained and is then *acted upon* is even more difficult. For this reason it is vital that, at the planning stage of projects, managers are given very clear responsibilities to meet specific objectives after the capital spending is over. Just as for IM&T projects, medical equipment, often highly computerized itself, must be managed to achieve the hoped-for benefits.

CONCLUDING POINTS

The business planning process can be applied just as easily to individual capital projects as it can to 'business' organizations. The benefits of capital projects have to be managed; they do not emerge while organizations wait passively for their rewards after the hard work of capital investment planning and implementation is over.

CASE STUDY 13   CAPITAL PROJECT OPTION ANALYSIS

Stovely NHS Trust

Stovely NHS Trust could make better use of its high quality new facilities if it could offer good transport facilities to patients in neighbouring areas. Significant extra numbers of people could be treated if efficient transport covering a radius of 50 miles from the Trust could be provided.

A business case is being drawn up which looks at both the revenue consequences of increasing patients and the costs, both capital and revenue, of providing transport. This case study looks at two key aspects of the mechanics of the cost–benefit analysis:

1. a benefits analysis using weightings.
2. the calculation of net present values (NPVs) for each transport option based on whole life costs.

The possible transport options being considered are:

- option A: do nothing;
- option B: contract with local bus company;
- option C: buy three minibuses;
- option D: buy one coach.

Benefits analysis

The Trust has identified five major benefits from high quality transport facilities for patients. They are listed below, together with a weighting that has been agreed after some consideration by the different members of the project team.

	Weighting (%)
1. Flexibility over patient numbers	30
2. Comfort of patients	20
3. No driver training required	15
4. Range of travel	25
5. Promotion of trust	10
	100%

Having agreed these weightings, the four options were scored by the project team. Scoring was out of 10. However, so that the weighting could be taken into account, the scorings were multiplied by the weightings. The results are shown in Table A.

Results of benefits analysis

From Table A it can be seen that option B, the contract with a bus company, had the highest weighted scoring. This option is therefore the favoured solution. However, at this stage the cost of the options have yet to be taken into account.

Table A Benefits analysis of patient transport options

Benefit	Weighting (%)	Option A Do nothing		Option B Bus contract		Option C 3 minibuses		Option D 1 coach	
		Score	Score × weight	Score	Score × weight	Score	Score × weight	Score	Score × weight
Flexibility over patient numbers	30	8	2.40	7	210	6	1.80	4	1.20
Comfort of patients	20	0	0.00	7	1.40	6	1.20	7	1.40
No driver training required	15	0	0.00	10	1.50	8	1.20	0	0.00
Range of travel	25	0	0.00	10	2.50	4	1.00	8	2.00
Promotion of trust	10	0	0.00	0	0.00	5	0.50	10	1.00
Totals	100	8	2.40	34	7.50	29	5.70	29	5.60

Calculation of cost of option C, purchase of three minibuses

In calculating the cost of this option 'whole life' revenue flows have been analysed as discussed in Chapter 8. These revenue flows have been subjected to discounting at 6%. Table B shows the calculation.

Table B Calculation of whole life costs discounted at 6% for Option C, purchase of three minibuses

	Year 1	Year 2	Year 3	Year 4	Year 5
Capital costs					
Purchase of three minibuses	72000				
Set up costs	1500				
Sale proceeds					−15000
Total capital	73500	0	0	0	−15000
Revenue costs					
Net income from 200 extra patients per week	−156000	−156000	−156000	−156000	−156000
Drivers	30000	30000	30000	30000	30000
Maintenance	7000	7000	8000	10000	10000
Licence and insurance	3000	3000	3000	3000	3000
Fuel	3500	3500	3750	4000	4000
Other services (estimated)	1000	1000	1500	1500	2000
Income from hirings	−1000	−1000	−1000	−1000	−1000
Net revenue cost/(saving)	−112500	−112500	−110750	−108500	−108000
Net cash flow	−39000	−112500	−110750	−108500	−123000
Discount factor 6%	1.0000	0.9434	0.8900	0.8396	0.7921
Discounted cash flow	−39000	−106133	−98568	−91097	−97428
Option net present value	−432226				

From Table B we can see that the NPV of the minibus option is £432 226. Similar calculations for the other options have been done, which give the following NPVs:

		NPV
Option A:	do nothing	0
Option B:	contract with local bus company	−291 023
Option C:	buy three minibuses	−432 226
Option D:	buy one coach	−401 297

Options B to D all show desirable investment returns. (Negative NPVs because income has been shown as a negative figure.)

On the basis of cost the best option is the minibuses. However, on the basis of benefits the best was the bus company contract. Which option, then, should be selected? Two issues need to be considered:

1. Cost–benefit analysis
2. Risk analysis

Cost–benefit analysis

Matching costs against benefits is in this case a subjective process. Is option B better than option C? This depends on whether the extra cost is worth the large number of extra benefits that B offers.

Risk analysis

If circumstances were to change then the benefits might change as well. In particular, in this case if the number of patients were to become certain then the effect of the 'flexibility' benefit would be significant. In the circumstances of signing a five-year contract with a purchaser the benefits analysis would change substantially. Table C shows the change. Option B is still the best but is still the most expensive. However, whereas the minibuses had marginally more benefits than the coach, now the coach looks the better option.

Conclusion

Option B, the bus company contract, has much the greater benefit even after the risk analysis has been carried out. It is a matter of judgement whether the benefits are worth the substantial extra cost or reduction in net income.

Table C Benefits analysis of patient transport options

Benefit	Revised Weighting (%)	Option A Do nothing		Option B Bus contract		Option C Three minibuses		Option D One coach	
		Score	Score × weight	Score	Score × weight	Score	Score × weight	Score	Score × weight
Flexibility over patient numbers	0	8	0.00	7	0.00	6	0.00	4	1.20
Comfort of patients	29	0	0.00	7	2.03	6	1.74	7	2.03
No driver training required	21	0	0.00	10	2.10	8	1.68	0	0.00
Range of travel	36	0	0.00	10	3.60	4	1.44	8	2.88
Promotion of trust	14	0	0.00	0	0.00	5	0.70	10	1.40
Totals	100	8	0.00	34	7.73	29	5.56	29	6.31

The minibuses (option C) give the best return or are the cheapest, closely followed by the coach (option D). The benefits analysis also showed the minibuses to be superior. On this basis the minibuses might be the preferred option – second best on benefits but the best financial deal. On risk analysis the situation reverses, and option D shows more benefits. Option D might be selected if the likelihood of a five-year contract was high.

This quantification of the issues regarding selection of the best option does not in the end remove the need for a subjective element in the decision process. However, it does help to clarify the issues so that a rational outcome becomes possible.

Key Learning Points

1. Project options require **formal analysis**.
2. Benefits from a project need to be **clearly defined** and recorded.
3. Benefits are not all of equal significance – they need to be **weighted**.
4. Costs need to be considered in terms of the **whole life** of the project.
5. Costs need to be calculated as **net present values** using a discount rate of 6%.
6. **Risk analysis** on benefits needs to be carried out.
7. Costs and benefits need to be **compared**.

Chapter 9

Private Finance Initiative

It is a central government requirement that major public sector capital projects need to be 'tested' in the private sector. This is to ensue that, where a private sector solution could be viable, it is properly considered. For this reason the Private Finance Initiative (PFI) will affect the business case process from the beginning.

WHAT IS THE PRIVATE FINANCE INITIATIVE?

In 1992 Kenneth Clarke, the then Chancellor of the Exchequer, introduced the idea of PFI. For major public sector capital projects the private sector should be approached to provide capital and take some of the risk 'which needs genuinely to be borne by the private sector'. In essence, he wanted to achieve two things:

1. Capital investment in the public sector without increasing the public sector borrowing requirement.
2. Privatization of large sections of the public sector.

Few politicians now contemplating power see in future a wholly publicly financed renewal of the country's capital infrastructure. For this reason, some form of PFI appears desirable to most politicians.

Since Kenneth Clarke's announcement, private companies have become increasingly aware of the money to be made from effectively building and operating major public assets. A big problem has been their limited experience and expertise in near state monopoly businesses such as hospitals.

Although there has been much to learn, the lure of major contracts in public sector businesses that are essentially very low risk has been effective. To help obtain the knowledge and skills they need, private companies have been forming consortia. In the health sector these will typically be composed of one or two service companies, a builder and possibly a bank.

HOW CAN THE PFI SUCCEED?

Many commentators have been puzzled about how a private consortium can finance and run a hospital, for instance, more cheaply than at present. Given that private sector capital financing costs are generally considered to be much higher than the government's cost of borrowing, this is a very reasonable question.

Three possible answers are often put forward, namely, *specialization, use of capital assets* and *low risk* in near-monopoly situations.

Specialization

Much of the public sector outside central government takes the form of an agglomeration of widely differing businesses. Local authorities are the most obvious example. They make policy, collect rubbish, operate sizeable housing businesses, pay state benefits etc. No private business would feel competent to carry on such a wide range of economically unrelated activities at this level, and none does.

In health the range of activities is not so large, but it is substantial – specialist refuse disposal, hotel services, cleaning, nuclear physics, specialist laboratories, professional medical consulting services, pharmacy, surveyors office. A chain of high street chemists would be happy running the pharmacy and possibly the hospital retailing. A major research company could perhaps look after the nuclear medicine. A hotel chain would understand the hotel services business. But none of these companies would expect to provide efficient world beating services if they had to carry on all of these businesses at once. For this reason commentators suggest that each element of the NHS is probably not as efficient or effective as a specialist company could be.

To external observers it is clear that more specializing on core businesses would strengthen the professionalism and efficiency of the activities that go to make up a health service. Of course, the issue arises as to whether each service in the NHS could be run by a separate business and still coalesce as a whole. The evidence to date is not clear cut, although contracted-out cleaning, catering and laundry have not caused major problems. Issues have arisen over the skills needed to manage contracts effectively. However, the evidence clearly does not prohibit an extension of the concept of health care as a partnership between separate specialist profit making businesses.

Use of Assets

The public sector has traditionally spent heavily on capital. For most private business major capital spending is something of a novelty, which is managed when the need arises. In the public sector capital investment is continuous.

This disparity between the investment patterns of the two sectors has led commentators to suggest that the public sector has many underused capital assets. Of course, this is not the public perception, which is often that there are too few. Any hospital closure is seen as a disaster, there are not enough council houses, and investment on the railways is 'non-existent'. In fact, many would suggest that both views are right! There are too many underused public assets and investment is too niggardly. Some assets, such as school buildings, are used from 8.30 a.m. to 3.30 p.m. for only 36 weeks a year. This represents usage for only 15% of the time. A factory working three eight-hour shifts and having a two-week Christmas break would achieve 95% usage.

Clearly, not every public asset can be used 95% of the time. Hospitals and clinics are probably used more than most private office space. Nevertheless, there is substance to the charge that health service assets are underutilized. Senior NHS estates management now holds this view publicly. And the more they do hold this view, the fewer of them there will be, so the evidence that they and their colleagues see must be exceptionally cogent! Obvious examples of underused assets are incinerators, car-parks and hospital equipment used for only a few hours or less each day. On top of underutilization there is waste. Space is wasted within hospitals, and equipment is purchased that is not compatible with other assets or is too expensive to maintain.

But how can hospital car-parks be used at capacity for more than eight hours a day, Monday to Friday? How can equipment be used for at least eight hours a day instead of for just a few hours a week. A car-park will be used more if it is well placed to service surrounding, perhaps non-health service, activities used out of normal working hours. So anything that can be done to achieve this will cut costs. Specialist equipment will have increased usage if it can be moved rapidly between sites. Lithotripter equipment is an obvious example where big savings have been made from portability. It is hoped and expected that large PFI schemes run by consortia of carefully chosen businesses will be able to site health service assets in advantageous ways to increase usage. More focused use of buildings and equipment should reduce waste.

Low Risk, near-monopoly situations

In 1995 the issue of pay for top management in privatized utilities resulted in the 'fat cats' debate. The public, via journalists, held the view that the main board directors of billion pound utility companies did not deserve the same pay as directors of other similar sized 'more competive' public companies. Part of the argument was based on an unwillingness to pay gas bills to 'subsidize' the lifestyles of managers. But the same view is not held regarding, say, the pay of international media stars. The key issue in the debate was in fact the issue of risk; where consumer choice is restricted, risk is generally lower.

Everyone needs gas, water and electricity. Providing these things is equivalent to organizing a beer festival in a brewery. The public perception was that the risks of failure are almost non-existent and if this is the case, why should the salaries be so high? This view is essentially correct as regards the old public sector monopoly businesses. It may not hold where the old utilities start to develop new businesses and markets overseas: recent examples include the failure of a major hospital project in Scotland. Whatever the rights and wrongs, the 'fat cats' debate does illustrate that most of the traditional health sector, and the wider public sector, is very low risk.

Despite a few examples of failure, in health the risk relative to most industries is clearly low. The service is largely a monopoly provided 'free' to the consumer but heavily rationed (choice is restricted) while being funded by the taxpayer. It is difficult to imagine a lower risk business. Because it is so low risk, it is highly attractive to profit making businesses. Capital will be attracted to a virtually risk free business, often guaranteeing long-term returns unaffected by recession. What could be more attractive?

We have explored some of the main issues that affect PFI. From these we can see that PFI is likely to remain and will probably grow in importance. It has 'intellectual' support from all major political parties, it makes good macro-economic sense and it tackles the issues of lack of specialization and underuse of assets in the public services. Its weaknesses are a lack of public support and little evidence of real achievement to date.

HOW DOES THE PFI WORK IN PRACTICE?

At the time of writing few large PFI schemes have come to fruition. Nevertheless, the forms in which PFI projects in the health service are now being formulated are quite clear. The options are as follows:

1. Design and build (D&B)
2. Design, build and finance (DBF)
3. Design, build, finance and service (DBFS)
4. Design, build, finance and operate (DBFO)

D&B is the first step on the PFI ladder. It is not, however, 'real' PFI because, although it transfers some risk to the private sector contractor, the finance remains public. This is no good to a Treasury that is strapped for cash.

DBF covers the weakness in pure D&B; the money comes from private companies. But those private companies will have to pay more for their capital than the government. DBF schemes achieve few of the specialization or use of capital benefits set out above, while the cost of money is higher than Treasury finance. These types of PFI schemes will normally fail on grounds of cost and value for money.

DBFS schemes are likely to be much more effective. Typically, in this arrangement a consortium of a property company, a construction company, a property services company and possibly a bank would attempt to put together a scheme that would benefit a range of potential players of which the NHS would be only one. Real benefits can now be obtained.

As an example, an NHS trust may wish to upgrade its existing buildings and construct a substantial new wing. A DBFS scheme could effectively achieve this by exchanging adjoining land for the work required. The consortium would use some of this land for the new wing and the rest for a commercial development complementary to the hospital. In addition, the consortium would continue to service the buildings regardless of user or owner for the medium to long term. Servicing would include cleaning, servicing of heating, air conditioning, water and electricity services as well as day to day and planned maintenance to the fabric of the building.

DBFO schemes offer more chance of cost effective solutions. The contractor or consortium will not only service the asset but also operate it. For a mobile lithotripter, this means that the hospital only has to provide a doctor. The equipment is provided, serviced and operated by a third party. In terms of NHS buildings, all support services could be provided by the contractor. This service could run from reception staff and porters through to carpenters and cooks. In the acute services of the NHS the vast majority of costs are property costs and nursing costs. Doctors and drugs account for only about 10–15% of the total. A DBFO scheme would therefore cover much of the costs of an acute service. It would not, however, include nursing or medical care services. Both of these are clearly NHS core business.

An area where there is currently much PFI interest is pathology. Services such as pathology, diagnostic radiology and pharmacy are not currently considered patient care and so can be subject to PFI. Such services represent about 10% of hospital costs so savings would be well worth taking. With pathology, for instance, many tests are very common and will be carried out thousands of times each year. Other tests, which may be quite simple, will only be required on a limited basis. For even a large general hospital to do these tests may be inefficient because most tests are highly automated. Any rare tests will have to be done manually at high price. Some less frequently used tests may cost only 20p each if automated but £100 each if done by hand. If tests such as these are done at a central location substantial savings will be achieved. PFI of pathology by a national operator theoretically makes such savings possible.

THE PFI PLANNING PROCESS

PFI, like all business planning, starts with an analysis of objectives. In NHS business case parlance the 'strategic context' needs to be clearly examined and recorded in a way that potential PFI partners will appreciate.

At the moment there are more NHS schemes than potential investors. This means that NHS bodies often need to *sell* their scheme to potential PFI partners, so there must be considerable additional planning above that needed for a 'normal' public finance investment. The additional planning will be carried out after clarification of the strategic context but before an outline business case is written. It is vital that the NHS body has thought through its needs and examined a range of possible ways of achieving that need, either by using public money or through a PFI route. In essence, at this stage a draft outline business case must be constructed as a tool for:

- clarifying logistical issues for the NHS body/Trust;
- sowing seeds of ideas into potential PFI partners;
- demonstrating to potential PFI partners that the NHS body/Trust has a coherent policy and is a professional and reliable partner.

At about the same time as this basic project planning is taking place, an advertisement will be placed in the *Official Journal of the European Union* (OJEU), announcing a major public sector investment is about to take place and inviting interested parties to respond requesting an information pack. At the moment many advertisements take the 'negotiated' route to public sector procurement for PFI projects. Select list or open tender options, as normally required through OJEU, currently appear too simplistic for many complex PFI projects.

Companies that respond to the advertisement will usually be sent an information pack, which, of course, needs to have been prepared before the advertisement is placed. Also important is the methodology for screening responding bodies after their presentation. Normally only three or four companies should be selected for negotiation. Weak unstructured screening is easily open to allegations of bias. There are many public procurement cases where such allegations have led to court cases.

TYPICAL STAGES IN A NEGOTIATED PFI PROJECT

Use of consultants

Where a major PFI project is planned an NHS body may well need consultants to assist. The main advisers will typically include:

- a major experienced firm of solicitors;
- a business/financial adviser;
- an architect or other building professional (for a building project);
- an equivalent professional for other project types (e.g. computer consultant, consulting engineer).

These advisers should ideally be engaged prior to advertisement or very shortly afterwards. Their skills will be needed as soon as the strategic context has been clarified and the decision has been taken to progress the project in some form.

Outline Business Case

Once the process has started to move forward the 'basic project planning' can be used to start to write the outline business case. Most of the work setting out the reasons for the investment will have been done. The work on the options will be prepared as required by the *Capital Investment Manual*, as will the assessment of costs and benefits and the risk assessment. A key issue here is the inclusion of (i) the 'do nothing' option and (ii) the in-house public finance option. These two will form the benchmarks against which PFI proposals will be tested.

Clearly at this stage PFI proposals will be limited to the initial ideas of shortlisted potential partners. The level of detail will be much less than that expected in a traditionally financed project. Rather than selecting a specific option as would normally be the case at this stage the document sets out, for the benefit of the NHS Executive:

- whether any investment should take place, and, if yes,
- what the PFI ideas are in outline, and
- the public finance benchmark against which they should be judged.

Negotiation and Selection of Partner

When the outline business case has been approved by the NHS Executive, negotiations with the shortlist of investors can be completed. At this stage all parties now know that a favourable outcome of some sort is likely. This is a big step forward.

At the negotiation stage of the planning, the three or four

interested investors submit ideas to the NHS body. At the end of this process each will give a price for their scheme. All of the schemes may be different so it is important that they are structured in a way that will allow comparison of costs and benefits. This will be done in the normal way for any NHS business case using discounted cash flows of whole life costs. Once the investor with the scheme that gives the best cost/benefit at reasonable risk and is cheaper than the public finance alternative has been chosen, the full business case will be produced by the NHS body and the investor in partnership. On approval of the full business case, work can start. Figure 5 summarizes the position.

POST-PROJECT IMPLEMENTATION

Once the project is operating it is crucial to manage the relationship with private sector partners. Skills in contract management are only being learnt slowly in the NHS. Errors in selecting and working with service contractors have been experienced by nearly every public sector organization. Only careful planning, care and constant vigilance will achieve the desired results.

When we discussed the potential benefits of PFI we said that increased specialization achieved by contracting-out could give benefits to the NHS. However, the risk was that the specialization benefits would be lost if all the disparate elements in a contracted-out hospital service could not mesh into a seamless whole. The key to success in this is, again, forward planning and strong management.

When services are contracted-out money must be kept back to manage the 'client side'. A manager working for the body that places the contract (the client) needs to be given clear responsibility for managing out the benefits of the contracted service for the benefit of patients. The manager must be knowledgeable, and responsible and must carry significant authority. All too often, such people are the managers that the contractor did not want to take when TUPE was applied ('Transfer of undertakings protection of employment': European law requires that when services are privatized the staff must transfer to the new contractor under their old conditions of employment).

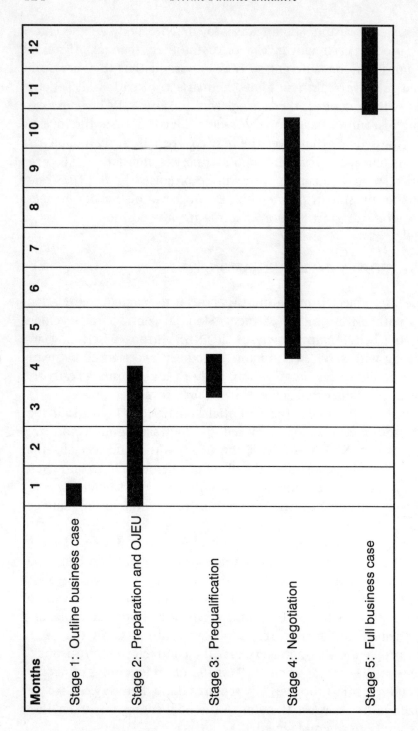

Figure 5 PFI procedures: a typical time scale

CONCLUDING POINTS

PFI is a complex process that requires professionalism. In particular, imaginative but thorough planning is important, covering:

- project outcomes;
- markets;
- senior management time and skills;
- future costs and income streams;
- post-implementation management.

Chapter 10

Implementation and review

COMMITMENT

The continuing nature of the business planning process is apparent from much of what has been said so far. This book supports a 'commitment building' approach to business planning. Harmonization of missions and objectives throughout the organization is a vital component of this approach. The case studies portray senior managers applying the business planning techniques in a way that enhances commitment at all levels.

A sense of 'ownership' is often critical to inspiring commitment: 'this is our plan and we want to make sure it works'. A sense of shared ownership reinforces the team spirit and, like all team building, tends to deepen a sense of commitment.

Sometimes it is easier to lead from the 'top down', convincing others of the value of your strategy and your vision of the organization's future. They in turn may come to regard this vision as embodying their objectives. Sometimes aspirations contributed from the 'bottom up' can revolutionize the mission of the organization, resulting perhaps in complete new services. When all of the high level strategies come from the top of the organization – a fairly common situation in practice – preparation from the bottom up is still worth while. Such preparation should take account of the nurses, doctors, managers, support staff and employees from as wide a range as possible. Few organizations of the size of a major hospital, and with all the diversity of functions it requires, can hope to coordinate and accommodate everyone's work-related aspirations. For example, broad conflicts between the desires for greater freedom of action and for greater job security and predictability will almost certainly have to be resolved at a senior level.

The critical point is that if large numbers of staff, or perhaps a few staff in key positions, feel that few of their work aspirations are embodied in the mission statements, objectives, targets or other aspects of the business plan then commitment to it will be a 'non-starter'.

Usually the most effective means of ensuring commitment is to draw out the high level statements from staff in a constructive and purposeful manner, then take these on board, perhaps with modifications but still recognizable by their original 'creators'. Giving staff at all levels the chance to carry out SWOT analyses, to be debated in staff meetings and 'quality circles' for example, is a well-known way of generating ideas and focusing attention on key issues and problems. Even if little of fundamental importance to the strategy and objectives emerges from this process, it will enhance a sense of commitment for many staff.

Ideally, though, such open discussions should lead to more concrete results. Initially these may well take a rather basic form of 'wish lists' or simple identification of common hopes and fears for the future. The careful business planner will mould these into supportive targets and objectives or possible services and improvements. If this cannot be done it is equally important to explain to staff why their efforts have been unproductive. Are they perhaps irrelevant to the agreed mission or incompatible with the needs of patients? In this way commitment building can become a learning process, which becomes ever more cost effective as time progresses.

It would be impossible to consider all of the potential influences upon, and ways of enhancing, a sense of commitment. In most situations a large number of activities and arrangements, each perhaps of little consequence in isolation, can collectively generate commitment. Some examples to prompt thought on this matter are given in Checklist 23.

Checklist 23

Examples of commitment-enhancing activities and arrangements

- Staff newsletter.
- Questionnaires to be answered (anonymously?), e.g. conditions of service, relevance of management targets to work undertaken, training needs etc.
- Regular staff meetings without any restriction on agenda, apart perhaps from time. Particularly important to aid commitment at a time of changing structures or management objectives.

- Quality circles and other more intensive group discussions or 'brainstorming sessions' to consider key aspects of the SWOT analysis.
- Achieving externally awarded quality and other standards such as ISO 9000 (BS 5750). 'Chartermark' or the Investors in People award.
- Internally awarded achievement standards, which can be particularly effective in larger organizations.
- Rumour countering, e.g. open and honest identification of threats and who gains or loses from proposed changes, access to information and clear identification of what has to be restricted and why.
- Rewards linked to the success of the business unit for staff at all levels.

Clearly one could continue the contents of Checklist 23. Each business planner will need to encourage activities that lend themselves to the services and the organization for which he or she is planning. Health service staff at each level tend to be relatively well educated, skilled and articulate. Any attempt to secure their commitment must recognize this. For example, blunt exaltations to accept the organization's commitments, blatant propaganda or 'company songs' are likely to attract well-deserved contempt.

REVIEWING, REPLANNING AND REORGANIZING

The success or failure of the business plan will need to be reviewed on a continuing basis. This will lead naturally into amending the plan, reorganizing and possibly restructuring the organization. Flexibility and adaptability are crucial as any plan must be able to accommodate the need for change. Although we have implied the superiority of continual review, review may be a more static stage of the planning process and still be effective in suitable circumstances. An example might be where previously agreed stages of capital works are of overriding importance to the business plan. The NHS Executive requires updated business plans each year. The temptation to provide the new year's plan by superficially rewriting the old one should be resisted!

Review will include financial, marketing, human resource and other information, as well as information from operational managers on their progress within the organization. It is essential that the review process can select, capture and utilize the appropriate contents of this 'feedback'.

It is virtually impossible to conceive of a situation in the health service where a business plan will remain relevant and unchanged indefinitely. The components of the plan, such as those outlined in Chapter 4, will typically require revision at least annually.

It is conceivable that high level statements may stand the test of time, lasting for many years, although even this is not common in such a rapidly changing, politicized environment as health care. It is inconceivable that service innovation and pricing decisions, for example, will not require frequent revision. The most dangerous temptation is to treat the compilation of a business plan as a one-off project to which lip service can be paid while everyone gets on with the job. Where this happens organizations are often characterized by a reactive 'crisis' style of management, with a lack of ability to meet competition and change.

As reviewing, replanning and reorganizing are repeated, established mechanisms will evolve if these have not already been built into the planning process. Herein lies another danger, although usually a lesser one than those so far considered: just as the plan cannot remain relevant indefinitely, neither can the channels of communication, procedures and events designed to shape it. The review procedure itself should come under review.

Many diagrams and formulae have been suggested to describe the planning and reviewing process. Often some form of circular arrangement is put forward with headings to represent the cyclical nature of the process. We are cautious of such all-embracing models. Business planning is perhaps a less systematic process than its name implies. The components of a plan can sometimes be usefully considered at almost any point, and the process can be started and worked on simultaneously at different points. Any of the components may be affected by a range of internal and external influences and hitherto less obvious links may rise to prominence. This very unpredictability needs to be recognized by planners. Nothing can be ignored indefinitely, nor will a predictable review process continue to cover all that is relevant. Figure 2 offered a very general overview but even this should be treated with caution.

CONCLUDING POINTS

The completion of a business plan or a business case for a particular project is the beginning of a continuing implementation process. The business planning process will be needed throughout the life of the organization.

CASE STUDY 14   MISSION, IMPLEMENTATION AND REVISION

Fitown Health Services NHS Trust

This case study examines the relationship between mission statements and management objectives under conditions requiring revision and change. This longer case is in four parts, as set out below. Much of the case, and the last part in particular, also relates back to Chapter 5.

1. Background. This sets out a brief overview of a typical NHS Trust.
2. Reviewing the *status quo*. Many NHS managers and others will recognize weaknesses highlighted by the original mission statement and lower level objectives. Managers have their own agendas and short-term concerns that are not fully focused on the corporate needs. The problems raised in this part of the case can apply to some extent in even the smoothest running organizations and departments.
3. Reviewing unit/departmental aims within the Trust. The emphasis here is on drawing middle and junior managers and clinicians into the process. Revised objectives are formulated for comparison with those in the second part.
4. Forging a new corporate mission. Senior management and directors ensure that the revised objectives and strategies are drawn together in a way that serves the interests of the Trust as a whole. A corporate mission and strategic objectives are agreed that are together greater than the sum of the parts, enabling clear improvement in the management of the Trust overall.

Background

The case is set in a Trust environment that provides a range of health services for one main purchasing authority, the Fitown and District Health Authority. The business units are arranged into central services units and operational services units. Figure 6 shows the structure of the Board of Fitown NHS Trust.

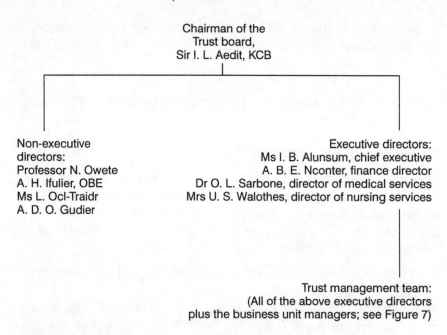

Chairman of the
Trust board,
Sir I. L. Aedit, KCB

Non-executive
directors:
Professor N. Owete
A. H. Ifulier, OBE
Ms L. Ocl-Traidr
A. D. O. Gudier

Executive directors:
Ms I. B. Alunsum, chief executive
A. B. E. Nconter, finance director
Dr O. L. Sarbone, director of medical services
Mrs U. S. Walothes, director of nursing services

Trust management team:
(All of the above executive directors
plus the business unit managers; see Figure 7)

Figure 6 Fitown NHS Trust board and management team

As well as being responsible for the operational business units run by the Trust, the chief executive and the executive directors are also responsible for the central services units. This means that they oversee both client and contractor roles involving internally traded services. Each operational and central service unit is headed by a unit manager. Figure 7 shows the unit management of the Trust.

Reviewing the *status quo*

The present mission statement of Fitown reads as follows:

'Fitown NHS Trust is dedicated to providing the highest possible quality of health care equally to all patients throughout all activities of the Trust. We aim to provide services efficiently in full cooperation with all other relevant agencies. We are committed to the promotion of high professional standards and to supporting all our staff in their training and professional development. The Trust recognizes the importance of honesty and clarity in all its communications.'

Irene Alunsum has recently been appointed as the chief executive. She is relatively new to the health service, having served

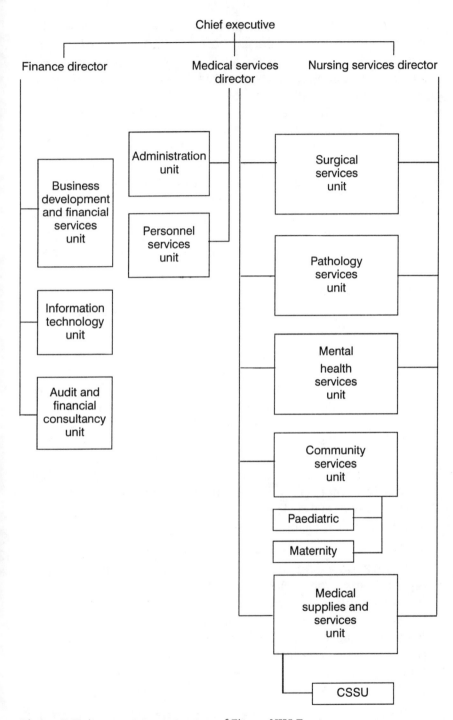

Figure 7 Unit management structure of Fitown NHS Trust

only a year as deputy to the chief executive of a nearby NHS Trust following a long career in the retail trade. One of the first tasks she sets herself is a review of the mission statement, with which she feels slightly uncomfortable. It seems, for one thing, to give cooperation with other bodies, and training – both very desirable means to an end – the status of ends in themselves. She also intends to review the management objectives contained in the current business plan. She considers herself to have fairly radical views on coordinating the management of diverse business units and devolving decision making. She is determined to put her ideas into practice while bringing other people on board.

The first meeting on the subject took place between Irene and Arthur Nconter, the finance director. In response to Irene's opening remark about the importance of a realistic business plan, Arthur commented:

> 'Of course, you'll have a hell of a job to get the board to take it seriously. They are, how shall I put it, well "traditionalists" is the polite term.'

'Surely they will see that the present plan is totally inadequate?' asked Irene.

Arthur suggested contacting the members of the Board to let them know about the intended revision of the business plan, reminding them of when it was actually prepared, to gauge their initial reactions. Irene did so, learning in the process that Arthur had been the main driving force behind the existing plan and that he was generally considered to be a meddling accountant. She was able to contact all of the Board members except Professor Owete, who was in the USA.

After further discussions with Arthur, Irene concluded:

> 'I think this will be a case of planning from the middle up and back down again. We will get the unit managers to report their current objectives as soon as possible, and use this to put the Board under pressure from above and below. I always feel it is best in the long run to construct the business plan around the business. I like as many people as possible, and all the business unit managers at least, to feel that the final mission statement is *their* mission, not something imposed on them by the likes of you and me.'

Arthur was a little surprised that Irene was able to refrain from simply attempting to stamp her own clear vision on the thing right from the start. He was sure that the unit managers were ready to follow any clear lead on this matter, and was not certain that this was going to be the right approach. Strong and unambiguous leadership had always been the hallmark of the past chief executives. For the moment he kept his concerns to himself. He wanted Irene to be right and rather liked the idea of a less autocratic approach, if it could be made to work. If nothing else, he told himself, we might get a few new ideas.

The following is a summary presented to Irene Alunsum of each main business unit and its corresponding management objectives, at the time of her appointment.

Surgical services

Although several objectives can be inferred from statements and the minutes of meetings, one clear objective stands out:

'To improve the operating infection rates by 50%'

This is stated as matching national averages. This department also includes an implied objective of reducing waiting lists for all classes of surgery and minimizing the number of cancelled operations. Few quantifiable targets have been set.

Paediatric Services

This business unit is made up of General Paediatrics and Special Care Paediatrics, and this is reflected in the management objectives.

General Paediatrics

The paediatric surgery undertaken has been set the same target as for surgery generally, although local management and paediatric consultants have agreed that they should better the national average, if this is known with certainty for any one year.

A Community Child Health Unit has recently been set up to work with the local authorities, schools and similar agencies in improving health and safety for all under-15s in the catchment area of the Trust. It has already adopted two objectives that form part of the 'Health of the Nation' targets, set as Government policy. The first of these, to reduce smoking among 11 to 15 year olds by at least 35% by 1994, has been stated by the unit manager as having been achieved, and less than 6% of children in this age group now smoke on a regular basis. The second, to reduce the death rate resulting from accidents among children under 15 by at least 33% by 2005, has yet to be achieved. There has been some criticism of the way in which the unit manager has measured the attainment of both targets.

Special Care Paediatrics

Plans are in hand to double the size of the intensive care unit for children to eight beds at the main hospital.

A target has been set to increase the survival rate of babies born weighing less than 1 kilogram by 20% over two years by setting up a special baby unit within the Special Care Paediatrics Division.

Mental Health Services

This is based at Fitown Psychiatric Unit, Little Pond Hospital, close to the Trust headquarters.

A code of practice, the Fitown Mental Health Care Code, has been established as an operational quality standard for all managers, and this includes a variety of key targets as well as recommended practices.

A 'Health of the Nation' target, to cooperate with other local agencies to reduce suicide rates in the catchment area by 10% within two years, has been formally adopted by the unit manager.

Finance Department

Three fairly well-defined departmental objectives have been set:

1. To balance the budgets over the medium term in line with directions from the board.
2. To meet or exceed the 6% rate of return on relevant net assets, as set by the Department of Health.
3. To remain within the current external financing limits (EFL) set by the Department of Health.

Several less firmly agreed objectives are implied within the department, including a detailed audit strategy that sets out a series of audits to be completed each year on an agreed basis with each responsible director.

The other main operational business units of the Trust submitted objectives that were considered by Irene Alunsum to be little more than restatements of the mission statement or of broad policy statements, rather than operational objectives capable of any practical measurement. On balance, the new chief executive was not greatly impressed with what was offered.

Reviewing unit/departmental aims within the Trust

Despite her concern at the efforts of the business unit managers, Irene Alunsum told herself that it was still early days. Nearly all of the statements related to periods over the past few years when little enthusiasm for planning existed at the Trust. Now Arthur, Professor Owete and the director of nursing services, Ursula Walothes, saw the importance of the business plan. Irene's aim was for the Board to give a lead in Trust business planning, spurred on by enthusiastic support from unit managers. The planning team agreed that the unit managers must be encouraged to be more proactive, even creative, and should examine their own business aims and what their operational aspirations really amount to. Looking at the planned changes from an accounting perspective, Arthur knew that he would have to get the unit managers to consider their budgets very carefully, but without discouraging their efforts.

On the next board meeting agenda Irene placed an item on the effectiveness of business unit objectives. She knew that this would not be as unpopular with them as a direct item on business planning. She wanted the board to develop a corporate strategy and mission statement from the aims and objectives of the units. At the same time, she knew that the board would not itself be able to produce these lower level strategies. Some of the board members were political appointees with little knowledge of the detailed problems of the units. In any case, there were too many issues for them to come to grips with in any reasonable time. But, most importantly, she wanted the units to feel they 'owned' their own strategies and that these were reflected in the corporate strategy and mission statement.

By this means, Irene hoped to avoid disharmony between the corporate mission statement and the main business objectives of each unit. At the same time, she felt that if the corporate mission is set without adequate understanding and awareness of each unit's desired business objectives then the chance to realign the units in the direction of the corporate mission (or amend the mission to accommodate the business needs of the units) would be unnecessarily hampered. 'Hidden agendas' will complicate the management of the organization as staff pay lip service to the mission statement and the 'imposed' management objectives while fulfilling the 'real' objectives. This problem may happen to some extent in any complex organization but Irene intended to minimize the risk as far as possible in the Trust.

For these reasons an effective forum for business planning was required below board level. Irene asked the business unit managers to arrange meetings of their unit management teams. She also asked for business planning to be included at their next Trust management team meeting. This was a senior management policy group, including executive directors, that met monthly.

Before the board meeting Irene asked each unit to consider its management objectives in whatever form these take and suggest 'mission statements' for its particular units. The unit managers were told that they should not feel constrained by the existing corporate mission statement of the Trust when drafting their suggestions.

The business unit managers were given two weeks in which to produce their responses for the relevant director and the Trust management team. The board meeting was set for two weeks after that. It is probably fair to say that some units would consider this a tight time scale as their managers have not been asked to work to specific objectives and have workloads that already place heavy demands on their time. Nevertheless, units and unit business managers generally welcomed the idea of influencing the board; it gave them a voice that they did not expect to have. In the two weeks available unit management meetings were held and considerable discussion within units took place. At the Trust management team meeting ideas were further refined.

After the Trust management team meeting 'unit mission statements' were put forward by all of the unit managers, and these were included with the board agenda papers.

We shall now consider three of these unit statements in more detail, those of the Surgical Services Unit, the Mental Health Services Unit and the Financial Services Unit of the Finance and Administration Department.

Surgical Services Unit, business plan period 1.4.97 to 31.3.02

The unit will continue to provide a wide range of general surgery and develop the existing specialist facilities in ear, nose and throat (ENT), trauma rehabilitation and plastic surgery relating to hand trauma and reconstruction.

The unit aims to continue as the single provider of these services to the Trust. Following the recent opening of a new surgical wing of the hospital no major expansion of this unit is foreseen during the current business plan period.

The unit aims to equal or exceed all national and local performance targets. *The unit will strive to maximize the quality of service in all respects within the resources available and ensure that it is always acceptable to patients and clients.* We are particularly conscious of the following key management objectives:

1. To improve the operating infection rates for each major class of operation to be within the top quartile of all Trusts.
2. To reduce waiting times after referral to a level where 80% of all referrals are seen within six months and 100% within nine months.
3. To be judged by the patient or his or her representative to have dealt appropriately with all accident and emergency admissions from the time of admission.
4. To contribute to the achievement of the corporate mission and goals of Fitown NHS Trust.

This mission statement is supplemented by a fully costed cash budget and a human resources budget. The chief surgeon is currently heading up a unit quality review team that also plans to produce a report on customer care and service quality.

Mental Health Services Unit, business plan period 1.4.97 to 31.3.02

The unit currently provides inpatient, outpatient and day patient mental health services. It also provides selected services to local authorities and voluntary bodies. The main facilities are based at Fitown and nearby Little Pond hospitals, including centres providing specialized support for carers of mentally ill outpatients.

The unit will maximize the quality of health care within the resources available and taking account of all relevant guidelines, including the Patient's Charter.

The unit intends to extend provision on a self-financing basis to other purchasers, without lessening its commitment to the Trust.

All services will operate within the Fitown Mental Health Care Code of Practice. The Code sets out guidance on mandatory and recommended best professional practice, deviation from which must be approved in writing at Trust board level by an executive director. The Code will reflect the needs and aspirations of service users, staff, carers and client bodies.

The first draft of the Code has been provided and procedural and quality systems manuals have both been started. A human resources budget based on approved staff complements and a cash budget on the income and expenditure estimates have also been prepared.

Financial services unit – business plan period 1.4.97 to 31.3.02

The unit's *overriding mission* is twofold:

1. To ensure the Trust has a sound financial basis from which to plan future activities and expansion.
2. To provide sound management information on which service managers can rely to manage and develop their businesses.

We are particularly conscious of the following key management objectives:

- To ensure that the Trust breaks even in the medium term.
- To provide a 6% rate of return on net relevant assets.
- To meet our external financing limits.
- To produce a balanced annual budget.
- To provide monthly management accounts to all budget holders and the board.
- To provide the annual accounts and report ready for audit by the first working day of June each year.
- To undertake a full range of planned internal audits and report to the audit committee of the board on a quarterly basis.

Appendices to this statement set out the staffing and cost implications of the statement.

For the sake of brevity, further examples of unit mission statements and their lower level management objectives have not been included in this case study. The issues they address follow the same pattern, with basic objectives, key targets and resource considerations set out.

In this particular organization no standard definitions of terms had been agreed. This is often the situation in organizations where business units have evolved along slightly different traditions and whose management structures reflect the uneven staff profiles needed to produce quite different services. It is frequently counterproductive to force a uniform terminology on such an organization, so long as each part of the business is clear about its own plans and the corporate management at board level appreciate any slight deviations in usage. In essence, this question revolves around the level of autonomy and separate management styles allowed to each business unit within the corporate whole. In this case study reasonably autonomous units are envisaged.

Forging a new corporate mission

The board meeting went well for Irene. She received much support from Arthur and Ursula and from Professor Owete, who does not often turn up for routine board meetings. The only opposition came from Dr Sarbone, who was concerned that consultants should have the maximum independence of action within each business unit.

Even Dr Sarbone's concerns were largely met by assuring him that units would continue to work very closely with consultants. As they will be taking decisions that affect other managers and consultants, it is vital that they do not work to conflicting objectives and, as far as practical, do work towards common corporate objectives. Set out below are some of the main points arising from the meeting.

Most of the key management objectives of the finance department are corporate-wide objectives, such as balancing the budget and meeting required rates of return, although the deadlines for achieving these act as key targets for this unit.

Commitment to quality is widespread among all units, with some working to achieve independent measures of quality assurance (ISO 9000 series and Investors in People).

Marketing efforts are at an underdeveloped level. Units perceive their role as no more than satisfying their main customer and accommodating minor secondary demands when these are placed upon them. There is very little proactive marketing.

Lack, or perceived lack, of a clear corporate mission statement has hindered each unit's own assessment of its impact on other units and the corporate whole. Examples of directly opposing management objectives between different units and objectives that are partly incompatible have come to light.

A need for more internal trading account information and income and expenditure forecasts was identified. Financial resourcing is generally inadequately covered compared with the detailed aims and objectives, although staff and equipment needs are usually well defined.

Much discussion ensued. The agreed choice was between a much more detailed mission statement or a short mission statement followed by a series of corporate management objectives designed to address the foregoing points. The later option was chosen.

The revised mission statement read:

'Fitown NHS Trust is dedicated to the highest quality of health care for all its patients. This care is to be provided efficiently, honestly and effectively by well-supported and highly motivated staff. To achieve this mission the following strategic objectives have been set for the next two years:

1. To identify at least one significant and practically realizable new source of income, or at least one significant increase in existing income, from each business unit.
2. To introduce a corporate quality policy based on the quality requirements and policies of all business units. This will include the phased introduction of total quality management strategy and the attainment of independent quality assessment to recognized international and national standards.
3. To undertake a corporate-wide review of management accounting procedures and the financial management information needed to improve the flexibility, awareness and preparedness of business unit managers to manage the resources at their disposal for the benefit of our patients.
4. To maintain a balanced budget while increasing the sources and total of income.'

The meeting drew to a close with all board members agreeing that a revised and detailed business plan was called for. The finance director was asked to chair a subcommittee for this purpose. Irene had succeeded in getting all of the important first elements of the business plan in draft form, had generated support and commitment from all of the unit managers and probably most of those working directly for them and, last but not least, has enthused her fellow directors with the need to undertake serious business planning rather than simply paying lip service to the latest fashionable buzz words.

Summary of case study

This case study dealt with high level aspects of business planning, providing an overview of potential problems. Perhaps the most critical point is that individual business units within the Trust must be allowed to develop business planning to meet the demands of their particular markets but this must be accommodated with the need for harmony with the corporate mission statement and objectives.

Compared to the private sector, such critical harmonization can be difficult to achieve. Corporate missions and goals can often be complicated by the unavoidable need to take on board local and national policies and wider social considerations. Added to this is the occasional difficulty of accommodating genuinely unusual market situations confronted by one or two units that cannot, for example, easily be sold off to other enterprises to allow the remainder of the Trust to concentrate on its core businesses.

In this case study the business units generally had some objectives related to quality, but prior to the revised mission statement and two-year corporate management objectives each unit had its own approach in isolation, leading, almost inevitably, to widely differing standards of care throughout the Trust. Similarly, marketing was poorly planned. It needed the impetus given by the corporate-wide objectives. At the end of the study the board aimed to draft a short but accommodating mission statement that was reinforced by, and gave leadership and direction via, its two-year high level objectives, which were in turn supported by the mission statements and objectives of each business unit. It did this not by bureaucratic coercion solely from the top down but by seeking opinions and offering leadership towards a common mission.

Key learning points

1. The business plan must be **revised regularly** to maintain its

relevance to all parts of the organization.
2. Any significant opposition, even at the highest level, **must be won over** if planning is to succeed.
3. The aims and aspirations of different parts of the organization must be **identified and harmonized** with a corporate strategy or mission.

Chapter 11

Some concluding thoughts

COSTS AND EXPECTATIONS

When the case in favour of a national health service was being most actively discussed following the end of the Second World War, one of the practical arguments often put forward was that it would lead eventually to an overall lowering of demand for health care as people became healthier. The population has indeed become healthier but the demand for care has spiralled. If it is not out of control, it is at least beyond any reasonable expectations of the time. Why is this?

Two main reasons have often been put forward:

1. Increasing expectations, as people have become more aware of the possibilities for treatment. This reason is bound up with some of the marketing aspects discussed previously.
2. Increasingly sophisticated technology and medical advances have opened up more possibilities for treatment.

It is only fair to point out that both of the above have given rise to and, to a lesser extent, been driven by, long-term expectations of increased government funding.

Marketing in the broad sense has a critical role to play in such expectations because knowledge about newly available treatments and availability of existing treatments often relies on formal or informal marketing.

HEALTH VERSUS HEALTH CARE

Marketing developments have been widely accused of concentrating too much upon the curative or treatment aspects, i.e. health care, rather than preventive policies, that is ones that promote health.

Selling cures to people who are ill, or complex and expensive remedies to those who treat them, seems more attractive than selling prevention. Prevention might well lead to a fall in demand for sales and treatment in the long run. If this scenario is indeed the true situation then the monumental rise in the costs of health care over the past few decades could be due, in some part at least, to the vested interests of producers, sellers and providers of health care. Will the widespread use of business planning make any difference?

If, as seems likely, the purchasers are motivated to spread limited budgets as far as possible, business planning can be of great benefit to them. The alternative is to spend in an unplanned or poorly planned manner, with lack of defined purpose or prioritization until the money runs out. At this point the issue becomes highly political, involving questions about total funding/taxation, about who should do the prioritizing and about how they should manage it. But two advantages of business planning are clear at this point: it provides a framework for value judgements and it helps senior managers to identify the need for major reorientation.

A framework for value judgements

Business planning can provide a measured framework in which value judgements about funding are linked to the mission statement and the supporting management objectives. Detailed costing of objectives and the methods of their achievement should be made easier within such a framework, because the full ramifications of the actions and how they affect other parts of the plan will be easier to identify, and consequently easier to cost. If resources are being wasted (from a purchaser's viewpoint) it will be easier to identify this.

Reorientation

Business planning makes it easier to identify the need for a large-scale shift or reorientation of high level objectives. Once identified, such a reorientation is easier to accomplish. Basically, this is because the planning process helps to clarify such needs. The advantage is by no means unique to 'business' planning. Rather, business planning can be particularly helpful in focusing attention on the financial and output-related implications, especially in relation to different business units, each of which may have different business priorities.

Taken together, these two advantages may help to overcome the issue of treatment versus prevention. If providers do indeed have a marketing and wider business philosophy that encourages production and sales of treatment rather than prevention, this will be more readily apparent, certainly to senior management. It may even be that the business plan will set its mission, quite openly, to maximize such sales in the anticipation that purchasers will be content to accept this.

If a 'covert' mission is undertaken to maximize sales of treatment while 'pretending' to look to prevention in the stated business plan, this will make such a plan very difficult to pursue, leading to increasing disharmony and poor operational trading results. If more and more managers are brought into the picture about the 'real' plan, then why bother to be other than open?

In practice, it is most likely that the purchasers will be looking to minimize costs within particular levels of effectiveness and quality, as governed by their own business plans. If preventive products and services can be shown to pay, i.e. be efficient over time, they will look to providers to provide these, and the marketing strategy that meets this demand will be the only one that can be accepted in a successful business plan.

No doubt there will be local anomalies; no doubt purchasers and providers will be able to continue in business, each missing the optimum balance between curative and preventive products and services. But for the balance to be continually and uneconomically weighted in favour of curative measures (or indeed preventive, although this is not the allegation) would require one, or a combination of, the following:

1. No effective business planning, or planning that pays little attention to the business interests of the purchaser or, in the long term, of the provider.
2. A large number of purchasers and providers effectively acknowledging that they are content to collude in favour of curative treatment to the detriment of prevention.
3. No effective split between purchasers and providers, combined with a monopolistic provision that favours cure rather than prevention.

A cynic might say that in the UK we have moved away from the last of these pitfalls but not yet avoided the other two. One of the purposes of this book is to help correct this weakness.

Index